When One Hour is All You Have

Effective Therapy for Walk-In Clients

When One Hour is All You Have

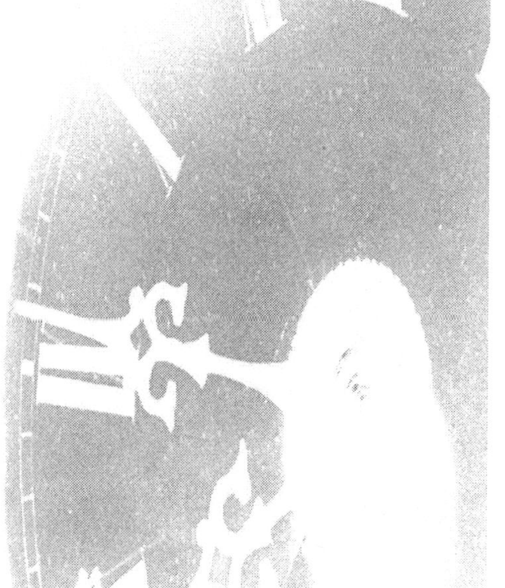

Effective Therapy for Walk-In Clients

Edited by Arnold Slive, Ph.D. & Monte Bobele, Ph.D.

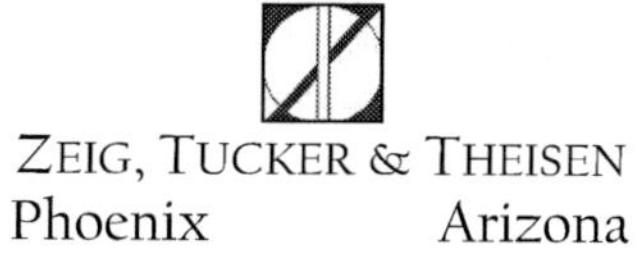

Zeig, Tucker & Theisen
Phoenix Arizona

Library of Congress Cataloging-in-Publication Data

When one hour is all you have: effective therapy for walk-in clients.
/ Arnold Slive, Monte Bobele — 1st edition.

p. cm.

Includes bibliographic references and index.
ISBN 978-1-934442-37-1 (alk. paper)
1. Counseling— mental health 2. Family—Psychological aspects.
I. Slive, Arnold II. Bobele, Monte III. Title

RC480.55.B77. 2010
616.89'14—dc21

Published by

ZEIG, TUCKER & THEISEN, INC.
3618 North 24th Street
Phoenix, AZ 85016

Manufactured in the United States of America

Contents

PART TWO
WALK-IN COUNSELING IN VARYING LOCATIONS

Acknowledgements

Although it may be trite to say it, this book would not have been possible without the help of many colleagues, students, and others.

Colleagues at Wood's Homes in Calgary (Chapter Six) had the courage to try something new and unusual in the face of potential criticism. Special thanks to those who were involved from the outset: Philip Perry, Jane Matheson, Susan Gardiner, Nancy McElheran, Ann Lawson and Harry Park and Margie Oakander. Thanks to the many clinical staff of Wood's, students and volunteers who helped us develop many of the ideas that are described in this volume.

Our Lady of the Lake University provided tremendous assistance for this project through the research resources of the Sueltenfuss Library and the funding of a graduate assistant to help with the completion of this book. The support and assistance of the faculty of the psychology department was especially helpful. Joan Biever, department chair, encouraged and supported this project from the very beginning. She read early drafts of some of the chapters and offered helpful suggestions. Bernadette Solórzano, Director of the Community Counseling Service, enthusiastically supported offering walk-in services at the CCS. Without opportunities to try out the ideas described in this book, we would have been unable to provide clear examples of our work.

Judy Larson, Dean of the Sueltenfuss Library, offered helpful advice at several stages of this project. She assisted in the preparation of the index and was a valuable consultant at several points in this project, especially regarding copyright issues.

Our collaborators in this project worked diligently with us through numerous requests for revisions of manuscripts. Our hats are off to them.

In many ways, the graduate students in the psychology department at Our Lady of the Lake were essential to the completion of this project. Several contributed case examples in Chapter Four. Two provided the excellent case example in Chapter Seven. Less conspicuous, but no less valuable, have been the student therapists who have worked with us on practicum teams in the CCS. Their questions, suggestions, and clinical creativity have been inspirations. They have helped to refine the ways we talk about brief therapy and the ways we have adapted our ideas to fit unique clients and contexts.

We would also like to recognize the advice and support that our colleagues Douglas Flemons and Bill O'Hanlon made early in the development of the book. Their ideas about content, potential contributors, and titles were helpful and encouraging. We owe thanks to Michael Hoyt for his encouragement and sage advice.

Monte owes a debt to Harry Goolishian and Glen Gardner for being mentors and role models.

With gratitude from Arnie to Susan, my best friend and inspiration.

Foreword

Michael F. Hoyt, Ph.D.

It is with great pleasure that I welcome *When One Hour is All You Have: Effective Therapy for Walk-In Clients*. The editors, Arnie Slive and Monte Bobele, and the contributing authors have done a fine job describing the history, theory, utility, and practice (clinical and administrative) of walk-in single session therapy. As one of the editors explained in an earlier article:

> Developed . . . as a result of community demands for greater accessibility to mental health services, walk-in therapy enables clients to meet with a mental health professional at their moment of choosing. There is no red tape, no triage, no intake process, no waiting list, and no wait. There is no formal assessment, no formal diagnostic process, just one hour of therapy focused on clients' stated wants. As well as meeting client needs, walk-in therapy is highly rewarding to professionals due to the simple fact that the clients' ability to access the service at their chosen moments of need without having to jump over multiple hurdles means that a large percentage are highly motivated. Also, with walk-in therapy there are no missed appointments or cancellations, thereby increasing efficiency. (Slive et al., 2009, p. 6)

The editors and their confreres very ably describe their particular methods, which dovetail nicely with the most frequently cited generic components of brief treatment (see Budman et al., 1992; Hoyt, 2009):

1. Rapid and generally positive working alliance between therapist and client.
2. Focality, the clear specification of achievable treatment results and goals.
3. Clear definition of client and therapist responsibilities.
4. Emphasis on the client's strengths, competencies, and adaptive capacities, which can serve to empower, engender hope, and invite a relatively high level of client participation.
5. Expectation of change, the belief that improvement is within the client's immediate grasp.
6. Here and now (and next) orientation, the primary focus being on current functioning and patterns in thinking, feeling, and behaving—and their alternatives.
7. Time sensitivity, making the most of each session, as well as the idea of intermittent treatment replacing the notion of a once-and-for-all definitive "cure."

It was at the Brief Therapy Conference held in San Francisco in December 1988 that my esteemed colleagues Moshe Talmon, Robert Rosenbaum and I first presented our own research (funded by Kaiser Permanente) on "Single Session Therapy: When the First Session May Be the Last." Operating from the assumptions that each session is a whole, potentially complete in itself; that the power ultimately is in the patient; that all you really have is now; and that helping people to make small changes can made a big difference, we found that, when given a choice, many patients were able to make significant and lasting changes after one session. These findings were reported in two well-received books (Talmon, 1990, 1993), numerous articles and book chapters (authored jointed and independently), and have been presented in workshops held throughout the United States and internationally. Noting that each case is unique, we described a series of clinical guidelines to facilitate the possibility of one session being adequate and sufficient:

1. "Seed" change through induction and preparation.
2. Develop an alliance by co-creating, with the client, obtainable treatment goals.
3. Allow enough time for the session to be a complete process or intervention.
4. Look for ways to meet the clients in their worldview while, at the same time, offering a new perspective or hope about the possibility of seeing and act-

ing differently.
5. Go slowly and look for the clients' strengths and resources.
6. Practice solutions experientially, using the session to help clients rehearse solutions, thus inspiring hope and forward movement.
7. Consider taking as time-out, a break or pause during the session to think, consult, focus, prepare, and punctuate.
8. Allow time for last-minute issues, to help clients have the sense that the session has been complete and satisfactory.
9. Give feedback, emphasizing the client's understanding and competency to make changes.
10. Leave the door open, letting the client decide if the session has been sufficiently helpful or if another session (or more) is needed.

It is interesting to see how well these suggestions hold up in *When One Hour is All You Have,* as well as the new directions and ideas the contributors and clients generate in their various and original ways. Client competency and empowerment are consistently emphasized as the different authors draw upon a variety of approaches—such as solution-focused, narrative, systemic, and hypnotic—that I have elsewhere (Hoyt, 1994a, 1996, 1998, 2000, 2001, 2009) referred to as *constructive therapies* to highlight their basis in social constructionist theory and to convey the connotations of positive, productive, and creative. Constructive therapies are based on the recognition that we are constructing, not simply uncovering, our psychological realities. How we make sense of our worlds—the stories we tell ourselves and each other—does a lot to determine our experiences, our actions, and our destinies. The authors of the volume in hand all endeavor to help clients look at their situations and themselves in ways that help them get "unstuck" and move forward in their lives.

Before turning to the exciting chapters that follow, please allow me to make a few additional comments.

1. *"Strike while the iron is hot" and "The readiness is all" meets "Be here now."* As my colleague Bob Rosenbaum wrote in one of our early papers: "My desire is not to see everyone for one session; my desire is to see everyone for one full moment, as long as that takes" (in Hoyt et al., 1992, p. 80). In a more recent letter to the *Monitor on Psychology*, he elaborates:

    > Dr. Talmon and I have recently altered our focus somewhat. Psychotherapy is not long or short; to view it this way sets up a false dichotomy. Psychotherapy depends instead on "good moments" where something profound shifts for a client. All the rest is preparation and consolidation. Because we feel psychotherapy needs to fo-

> cus more on these critical incidents of change, we no longer talk of "single-session therapy" but prefer, instead, to examine 'therapy moment by moment' (Rosenbaum, 2008, 4).

I agree, but prefer to retain the catchy term *single-session therapy* because it emphasizes the idea that therapy can happen in "one hour," as well as to maintain continuity with existing literature.

2. *One at a time.* This is not to say that clients necessarily should only be seen once. It simply says we should not assume that more sessions would be required. The choice of whether to have more meetings usually is best left to the client. Put simply, there are essentially three ways to have a single-session therapy: (1)client stops unilaterally—often called "no shows" and "premature termination"—if the therapist is not open to the possibility that one session can be adequate and sufficient; (2)therapist stops unilaterally—usually only if the patient is poor and can't pay or can pay but is too difficult or challenging to make it appear worth continuing; or (3)client and therapist mutually agree that the one session has been enough—at least for now. Obviously, the third is generally the best. The work should not feel frantic or pell-mell; introducing the possibility of one-session being enough concentrates the mind and sets expectations that something will happen. Longer involvement should be available for those who need long term therapy, and doing very brief therapy with many folks will conserve resources for those who need them. Also, knowing that they can come for a single visit and not be obligated (read: trapped) can serve as a way for people both to access help and to enter the larger system, if more services are needed and desired.
3. *The importance of expectations.* As Stephen Appelbaum (1975; also see Battino, 2006) noted in his paper, "Parkinson's Law in Psychotherapy," clinical work often expands or contracts to fit the time allotted. In the original single-session therapy project that my colleagues and I did at Kaiser in the 1980s, patients came to the Psychiatry Department expecting an intake interview and approximately half got the help they needed in one visit. In *When One Hour is All You Have* clients usually came to the walk-in clinic expecting a self-contained episode in which something would get accomplished in the one visit. As editors Slive and Bobele note in their Introduction, the walk-in approach is an especially good fit for clients who have become accustomed to other walk-in services: church confessionals, government offices, barbers', beauty shops, and garages. Extended therapy, in which intake procedures must be completed before prolonged therapy can begin, may be something of a middle-and upper-class notion—although as our Kaiser experience showed, many clients can and will utilize one ses-

sion if given the choice. Along related lines, Jay Haley (1969, p. 76), in a paper in which he sarcastically mocked ways to endlessly extend therapy, advised ignoring the real-world problems of patients in favor of discussions about their infancies and inner-life fantasies, and added: "Avoid the poor because they will insist upon results and cannot be distracted with insightful conversations."

4. *Psychohealth, solution, and partnership.* As Moshe Talmon wrote in his fine 1993 book, *Single Session Solutions*: "These concepts represent an alternative to the traditional model in psychiatry and psychotherapy: psychohealth replacing psychopathology, solutions replacing problems, and partnership replacing patronization, domination, and hierarchy" (p. 73). Working the way we and the contributors to *When All You Have is One Hour* like to work —drawing from a variety of approaches that privilege clients' ways of knowing and competencies to help them achieve outcomes they define as successful—can entail a collision of several paradigms that upsets the psychiatric-industrial complex: Who's in charge here? Whose therapy is it? Who really holds the keys and the power? And how do you make a lot of money if they only come one time? To my mind, focusing on and working with clients' strengths and resources, their personal theories of change, values and worldviews is in the best spirit of Milton Erickson's (Haley, 1973; Short, Erickson & Klein, 2005) competency-seeking ideas about *utilization* and also fits nicely with evidence that it is the client's (not therapist's) contributions that most influence good outcomes(Miller et al., 1997; Duncan & Miller, 2000). Alas, as my colleague Steve de Shazer once cogently quipped in an interview, when discussing the difficulty of getting many trained clinicians to focus on clients' strengths and abilities: "[T] hey're not 'mental health,' they're 'mental illness' professionals. It's not a mental health industry; it's a mental illness industry" (Hoyt, 1994b, p. 20). The view that we prefer is optimistic, respectful, resource-focused, and pragmatic.
5. *"What's good for the goose...."* Clients sometimes come in with the expectation that a meeting will yield some sort of process and result that will not necessarily "cure" them or completely solve a problem but nonetheless will be of help to them. I recall an incident during our original Kaiser single-session therapy study during which I realized something valuable. We were consulting by phone through a one-way mirror. I discovered that it was often more helpful if we tried to align ourselves with the therapist's intention—making suggestions to help whoever was the therapist to do what they were trying to do—rather than reframing and redirecting the whole enterprise into our pet theories and making suggestions that jerked the process around to fit where we wanted to go. I thought about it some,

> then realized that there was a parallel process going on: The therapist did better with the patient, just as we did better with the therapist, when we supported the other person's intention and worldview.

This seems to me a very respectful way of appreciating diversity, attempting to learn from and work with whatever the client brings to the situation.

Currently, insurance companies, health maintenance organizations, clinics, counseling centers and consumers themselves all desire, and often require, brief treatment for psychological problems. Moreover, healthcare reform will open services for more people, perhaps creating democratic and cost-effective delivery systems where people can walk in and meet with a mental-health professional when they are ready. This is what many people want, need, and benefit from. True to Jay Haley's comment (Talmon, 1993, flyleaf) that "We once assumed that long-term therapy was the base from which all therapy was to be judged. Now it appears that therapy of a single interview could become the standard for estimating how long and how successful therapy should be." *When One Hour is All You Have* gives readers much to consider and apply. I am grateful to editors Arnie Slive and Monte Bobele and the other contributors for this fine volume.

References

Appelbaum, S.S. (1975). Parkinson's law in psychotherapy. *International Journal of Psychoanalytic Psychotherapy*, *4*, 426-436.

Battino, R. (2006).*Expectation: The very brief therapy book*. Norwalk, CT: Crown House.

Budman, S.H., Hoyt, M.F., & Talmon, M. (Eds.). (1992). *The first session in brief therapy*. New York: Guilford Press.

Duncan, B.L., & Miller, S.D. (2000) *The heroic client: Doing client-directed outcome-oriented therapy*. San Francisco: Jossey-Bass.

Haley, J. (1969).The art of being a failure as a therapist. In *The Power Tactics of Jesus Christ and Other Essays* (pp. 69-78).New York: Avon.

Haley, J. (1973).*Uncommon therapy: The psychiatric techniques of Milton H. Erickson, M.D.* New York: Norton.

Hoyt, M.F. (1994a). (Ed.) *Constructive therapies*. New York: Guilford Press.

Hoyt, M.F. (1994b). On the importance of keeping it simple and taking the patient seriously: A conversation with Steve de Shazer and John Weakland. In M.F. Hoyt (Ed.), *Constructive Therapies,* (pp. 11-40). Reprinted in M.F. Hoyt (2001), *Interviews with Brief Therapy Experts* (pp. 1-33). New York: Brunner-Routledge.

Hoyt, M.F. (1996). (Ed.) *Constructive therapies* (Vol. 2). New York: Guilford Press.

Hoyt, M.F. (1998). (Ed.). *The handbook of constructive therapies.* San Francisco: Jossey-Bass.

Hoyt, M.F. (2000). *Some stories are better than others: Doing what works in brief therapy and managed care.* Philadelphia: Brunner/Mazel.

Hoyt, M.F. (2001). *Interviews with brief therapy experts.* New York: Brunner-Routledge.

Hoyt, M.F. (2009). *Brief psychotherapies: Principles and practices.* Phoenix, AZ: Zeig, Tucker & Theisen.

Hoyt, M.F., Rosenbaum, R., & Talmon, M. (1992). Planned single-session psychotherapy. In S.H. Budman, M.F. Hoyt, & S. Friedman (Eds.), *The First Session in Brief Therapy* (pp. 59-86). New York: Guilford Press.

Miller, S.D., Duncan, B.L., & Hubble, M.A. (1997*). Escape from Babel: Toward a unifying language for psychotherapy practice.* New York: Norton.

Rosenbaum, R. (2008). Psychotherapy is not short or long. *Monitor on Psychology,* 39(7), 4, 8.

Short, D., Erickson, B.A., & Klein, R.E. (2005*).Hope and resiliency: Understanding the psychotherapeutic strategies of Milton H. Erickson, M.D.* Norwalk, CT: Crown House.

Slive, A., McElheran, N., & Lawson, A. (2009). How brief does it get? Walk-in single session therapy. *Journal of systemic therapies*, 27, 5-22.

Talmon, M. (1990). *single session therapy: Maximizing the effect of the first (and often only) therapeutic encounter.* San Francisco: Jossey-Bass.

Talmon, M. (1993). *Single session solutions: A guide to practical, effective, and affordable therapy.* Reading, MA: Addison-Wesley.

Introduction

Arnie Slive, Ph.D. and *Monte Bobele, Ph.D.*

Walk right in and sit right down,
daddy, let your mind roll on.
You'd better walk right in and stay a little while,
daddy, you can't stay too long.
Now everybody's talkin' 'bout your new way of walkin',
Do you wanna lose your mind?
Lord, walk right in and sit right down,
daddy, let your mind roll on.
— *Cannon/Woods (1929)*

Two Stories

Arnie

In the late 1980's, I was the Clinical Director of a large non-profit agency that provided a wide range of services for adolescents and their families. The agency is Wood's Homes and is located in Calgary, Alberta, Canada. One of the services we offered was outpatient family therapy. Families that were referred to that service were first asked to fill out intake forms, then meet with an intake coordinator, and if deemed appropriate for the service, were placed on a waiting list. If the length of a waiting list can gauge success, this was a very successful program. However, as the waiting list grew, we had more and more questions about the effectiveness of the service. Basic survival issues challenged many of the families we saw. Some were new to Canada, many were led by struggling single parents or were on the edge of poverty. Violence in the home was not uncommon. A high percentage were involved with child protection services. By the time a family got to the top of the waiting list and was contacted to make an initial counseling appointment, months might have passed. Sometimes the parents had forgotten they were on the waiting list or why they had contacted us in the first place. Often, they made an appointment and did not show up. Sometimes they showed up more out politeness than a sense of current need.

We began to ask ourselves if this was the best way to organize a service. So we went to the community and asked for feedback. We asked other mental health service providers, educators, political representatives, and volunteer community leaders. (Calgary was formally divided into communities with each community electing volunteers to run its association and represent them to the city). The most valuable feedback came from those volunteer leaders. From their perspective, based on their perceptions of the needs of the community, mental health services were, at best, inaccessible. At worst, they were irrelevant. For example, it was during this time that the Calgary newspapers reported in a front-page headline that the public schools were planning to cut back staff. Two of the groups targeted for cutbacks were school psychologists and English-As-a-Second-Language (ESL) teachers—those who provided specialized educational services for children of new immigrants. In the succeeding days, there was uproar about the potential loss of ESL teachers, but nary a word was said about the loss of school psychologists. In my view, the psychologists were providing a valuable service, but it was largely hidden from public view. Most citizens were unaware of the work of these valuable professionals.

The local agencies that offered counseling, like our own outpatient family therapy service, had similar problems—long waiting lists and cumbersome intake processes that included lengthy assessments. After searching through numerous alternatives at Wood's Homes, our executive director, Dr. Philip Perry, proposed a solution to the inaccessibility problem: eliminate the need for an appointment. I was assigned the task of making that a reality.

In 1990, we launched the Eastside Family Centre (EFC) (Chapter Six) and closed our more traditional outpatient family therapy program. EFC addressed the problem of inaccessibility by reducing the hurdles to be seen by a therapist. Six days a week, clients could come without an appointment and have a one-hour therapy session. There was no fee. There was no assessment. There was no screening. Whoever walked in, individuals, couples, or families, got a session that addressed the need(s) identified by the client(s).

I remember the first walk-in client I saw, not so much for the issues discussed as for the gratitude expressed by the client at the end of the session. Her gratitude was not for any specific help I offered; it was for the opportunity to have a conversation with a professional at a time that was most meaningful to her.

From the beginning, the idea of walk-in/single sessions did not seem like a stretch to me. Like Philip Perry, I was influenced by the work of Milton Erickson who was well known for his many single session case examples. Other influences included Mental Research Institute (MRI), Jay Haley's strategic approach, the brief approaches of the Milan Team and many other family systems models. I had begun to understand in graduate school that meaningful and long-lasting change can begin by taking one small step, and each of these influences supported that idea.

In 2007, Susan and I moved to Austin, Texas to be close to our grandchildren. That put me within a relative stone's throw of San Antonio and the work that Monte and his colleagues were doing at Our Lady of the Lake University. They were kind enough to let me walk right in. Monte and I have been collaborating ever since.

Monte

My interest in walk-in/single-session work developed along a different path. My journey began with a fascination with brief forms of therapy. I was in graduate school at a time when behavioral forms of therapy were beginning to supplant psychodynamic therapies. These behavioral interventions regarded long-term explorations of the unconscious as inefficient and offered behavioral alternatives that were considerably less time intensive.

I agreed, to some extent. I was embarrassed by my profession's reputation for inefficient long term therapy. For example, this stereotypical interchange between Woody Allen and Diane Keaton in *Annie Hall:*

Annie Hall: Oh, you see an analyst?

Alvy Singer: Yeah, just for fifteen years.

Annie Hall: Fifteen years?

Alvy Singer: Yeah, I'm gonna give him one more year, and then I'm goin' to Lourdes.

In the 1970s, Bob Newhart played a private practice psychologist, Dr. Robert Hartley, on a long running CBS sitcom. One of the recurring gags was a patient who came in week after week to Hartley's office and never said anything. Bob continued to schedule weekly appointments. Finally, in one episode, in frustration, Hartley shouts "What the heck do you want?"

I was also fascinated with accounts in the learning literature about single-trial learning. For the most part, descriptions of single-trial learning were accounts of classical conditioning like taste aversions and avoiding hot stoves. But there were others. For example, nearly every psychology student encountered the famous drawing of the young woman and the old crone. Upon encountering this ambiguous drawing for the first time, the viewer sees either an old woman or a young woman. Interestingly, the nature of the ambiguity prevents the observer from simultaneously seeing both figures. With some instruction or hints, however, the observer can usually easily see the second figure. Now, I have used this drawing, over the years, in various classes and workshops as an illustration of a number of psychological principles. I have been struck with the fact that regardless of how many years have passed since a student's or workshop attendee's first encounter with this drawing, they can easily make out both figures. The ambiguous effect remains with them, long after the first, and usually only, learning experience they had with the figure. This phenomenon led me to conclude that perceptual/cognitive learning can also take place in a single session and have permanent, lasting effects. The learning that takes place in this instance is not dependent on reinforcement. Observers rarely have difficulty spotting both figures, even if the learning took place many years earlier. There are a number of optical illusions that are like this.

I was also interested in the psychodynamic theory that a single traumatic event could produce permanent or relatively permanent neurosis in an individual. I began to think it might be at least logical that, if a single healing event could produce long-term psychological consequences, then perhaps a single traumatic event such as psychotherapy can produce long-term counter-pathological effects on clients. It also seemed important to remember that the longer a person might be in therapy, the more likely the therapy itself might become the problem rather than the solution. In classical psychoanalysis, it is axiomatic that the presenting problem is simply epiphenomena of some deeper, more profound problems. Since the nature of these conflicts was unknowable, the psychoanalytic approach required the establishment of a "transference neurosis." Apparently the features of a transference neurosis were knowable, and thus treatable. The elimination of the transference neurosis was the goal of therapy. The disappearance of the original troubles accompanied the elimination of the transference neurosis.

Early in my career, I was also aware of the literature showing that most therapeutic gain takes place the first few sessions. Many studies over the years have shown that although there is some slow gradual improvement after eight to ten sessions of therapy, the changes are small and almost inconsequential.

So it seemed that the therapy itself could become the problem the longer it lasted.

My own observations of therapeutic progress in my private practice, early on, were discouraging. I started out in a well-established practice that had a dozen full-time therapists and an extremely busy waiting room. Some people had been clients of the psychologists for many years, even for a couple of decades. In some cases we were seeing two or three generations of the same families in therapy. Progress was slow. That's what the textbooks told us. That's what we told one another, and that's what we told discouraged clients.

I eventually discovered the Galveston Family Institute (GFI) and its team of innovative, unconventional thinkers and therapists. Galveston was only an hour south of my home in Houston, and I began training with them, commuting there once a week. And the end of the first year, I arranged to complete a post doctoral training year with them. Harry Goolishian, George Pulliam, Lee Winderman, and Harlene Anderson were significant contributors to my theoretical and clinical development. GFI was influenced by the MRI and its Brief Therapy Project and the Milan therapists who developed a ten-session model for working with severely psychotic families. I learned early that most family therapists operated from a brief-therapy position and had invented theories to explain and prescribe brief therapeutic practices.

We appreciated many of the cases from GFI from this perspective. That is not to say that some cases were not long term. Harry used to remind us that he continued to see a man and his family that had he had begun with in the early '50s. Harry explained that this client contacted him periodically for a consultation and sometimes years would go by between consultations. Harry explained his perspective on therapy this way: "When you have a headache, you take an aspirin. You don't expect that one aspirin to cure headaches for the rest of your life. New headache, new aspirin." Minuchin has been known to describe his relationships with families as similar to the family doctor. The family doctor is a professional that the family consults as needed. Different issues may arise that require a new visit. So, for Minuchin, each treatment episode was a self-contained course of treatment. With single-session work, we strive to make each visit a self-contained treatment episode.

When I eventually left Galveston, I joined the faculty at Our Lady of the Lake University (OLLU) in San Antonio. So, when I arrived in San Antonio, it seemed to be a perfect context to continue training and treatments in brief therapies. OLLU had a fledgling family therapy program and a small clinic that provided a practicum experience for the graduate students. The university was located in a poor, Latino neighborhood. The prospective clients were not interested in long-term commitments to therapeutic conversations. They were people who saw therapy, or counseling, as a means to a relatively quick resolution to their problems. For the most part, they were not interested in self-exploration, personality reconstruction, or other long-term projects. Our clients wanted their adolescent children to do better in school and be more respectful. They wanted their spouses to listen to them, demonstrate caring, and take out the garbage. My interest in brief therapy and training others in brief techniques had found a home.

As I reflect on the cases that stand out, without a doubt, many of them were cases that were seen for 10 or more sessions. But, for the most part, my own clinical experiences have been with cases that needed five or fewer sessions. Twenty years ago, I published a paper about brief therapy in life-threatening situations. That paper described two cases: one involving domestic violence where the client's life had been threatened, the other a young adolescent who had just lost a prematurely delivered baby and who had made death threats against one of the house mothers in the home she was living in. Both of these cases reached a resolution by the end of the first session. I learned from these cases that unexpected changes are possible in a relatively short period time.

So, the fortuitous accreditation visit to Calgary in the early 1990's, where I met Arnie and saw the implementation of a walk-in clinic that focused on brief therapies, inspired me to develop something similar here in San Antonio. There were a number of institutional and contextual factors that prevent a wholesale transplantation of the Eastside Center's practices to San Antonio. However, we have incorporated many of the ideas. Our implementation is described in Chapter Seven. I am thrilled that circumstances have come together so that Arnie has become an integral part of our training and teaching program at OLLU.

Part One
Overview and Basic Principles

Chapter 1

WALKING IN: AN ASPECT OF EVERYDAY LIVING

Arnie Slive, Ph.D. and *Monte Bobele, Ph.D.*

You can get anything you want, at Alice's Restaurant.
You can get anything you want, at Alice's Restaurant.
Walk right in it's around the back,
Just a half a mile from the railroad track.
You can get anything you want, at Alice's Restaurant.

—*Arlo Guthrie, 1967*

We live in a fast-paced culture. Schedules are tight, meetings and appointments get squeezed into ever narrowing time frames. In this environment, there are times when it isn't possible to plan ahead and make an appointment. The business world has adapted by developing services that are immediately accessible without a pre-arranged appointment. Hence, we have fast food, drive-in banks, walk-in hair stylists, "no appointment necessary" income tax services, "just in time inventories," and even walk-in wedding chapels. The same is now true for medical clinics. Patients walk in and see a doctor without an appointment. If they return, they may see the same or a different doctor, though the next doctor will review the record from prior visits and take those visits into account in the current visit. Many dental and veterinary practices also encourage walk-ins. Church confessionals are usually conducted on a walk -in basis. The "Walk-ins Welcome" philosophy is so common because fits our lifestyles. This begs the question: What about walk-in mental health services?

Walk-In, Single-Session and Brief Therapy

Walk-in therapy and single-session therapy are forms of brief therapy. Brief therapy approaches have developed extensively over the last several decades. These models challenge the idea that enduring change must come through long and laborious mental health interventions. There is consistent evidence of the remarkable effectiveness of brief interventions in the literature. It is consistently reported that most client change occurs during the initial sessions of the therapeutic encounter (Chapter Two). There are many schools of thought ranging from psychodynamic to systemic to behavior therapy that have influenced the development of brief therapy models (Hoyt, 2009). All are based on the idea that change can occur in relatively few sessions. Post-modern, social constructionist, systemic and Ericksonian ideas influence this approach. Nevertheless, we strongly adhere to the notion that any model of therapy can be adapted to walk-in work provided that there is a strongly held belief that a whole therapy can occur in one hour and that a single hour of therapy can lead to significant change, even for longstanding issues.

Walk-in therapy is both similar to and different from single-session therapy (Talmon, 1990). Both treat each session as a complete therapy, in and of itself. In both approaches, clients present a concern and goals are constructed. Both aim for clients to leave with a sense that they've been heard, with hope, and with an increased awareness of their strengths and resources. In some circumstances, clients may have also begun to develop a plan on how to address their issues by the end of the session.

The most obvious difference between the two is that single-session therapy requires no appointment—clients just walk in. Likewise, walk-in services invite clients to return as often as they choose, on their own schedules.

Walk-in counseling is not new, nor is it solely a North American phenomenon. The oldest walk-in counseling service that we know of started in Minneapolis in 1969 and was influenced by the free clinic movement in California in the 1960's (Chapter Five). Beyond the United States and Canada, walk-in mental health clinics exist in England, Ireland, Australia, Israel, Jamaica, Zimbabwe and other countries.

The Case for Walk-in Counseling

In Chapter 2, we will present the research evidence that supports the concept of walk-in, single session therapy. To briefly summarize that evidence:

- Most therapy is brief therapy, whether by design or happenstance. The modal or most frequently occurring number of session in all models of therapy is one.

- The rate of change over the course of therapy decreases as the number of sessions increases. Most change occurs in the earlier sessions.

- Brief therapy has been proven effective.

Beyond the research about the relative brevity of therapy, we suggest that there are a number of other reasons for considering the development of walk-in services:

- Most clients want therapy to be as brief as possible. Many of the clients who come to Community Counseling Services (CCS) in San Antonio (Chapter Seven) expect to come for only one session. They expect that the session will work for them. Often, it is the therapist, not the client, who believes that therapy should continue with additional appointments. When therapists suggest an additional appointment at the end of the session, some clients seem surprised, disappointed, and discouraged. Frequently, clients who make a second appointment do not appear for the next session. The therapists are then surprised, disappointed, and discouraged. After all, based on both therapist perception and client feedback, the first session seemed to go well. But, the fact that the first session went well may indeed be the reason the client did not return. So mental health professionals have a choice. We can try to fit our clients into the traditional belief that therapy is a protracted process, perhaps many sessions over months or even years, or we can adapt what we do for the many clients who prefer one or a few sessions. A walk-in, single-session service is one way to address the wants and needs of some of our clients.

- In order for a client to receive treatment in many counseling agencies several steps may be required. Typically, a prospective client phones to inquire about setting up an appointment. The agency then asks the client to go through an intake process. That process may involve the completion of several forms and, perhaps after a period of waiting, meeting with an intake coordinator. The client may have to return for their first session with a therapist following that intake appointment. That first session (or sessions) may be considered an assessment. Only after the assessment does the actual therapy begin. Adding to the problem, the length of time from the initial phone call to the beginning of therapy will vary depending on the length of the agency's waiting list. The time period could by anywhere from a few days to many months. It is easy to see how clients may become discouraged or intimidated by this process and lose any motivation they had for therapy.

In contrast, a walk-in service does not even require a phone call. The only steps are to show up, fill out a brief form, and wait for the session to start. There is no screening; anyone who shows up is seen. The first session is not an assessment; it is a session of therapy. If clients want more sessions, they can show up again in the same way and as often as they like. In a review of length of therapy research (Barrett al., 2008) we learn that 50% of prospective clients who make an initial phone call to a public mental agency do not follow through with the initial intake meeting. If a walk-in service were available to them, how many of those callers would become actual clients?

- One of the advantages of a walk-in service is that it allows clients to access counseling at their chosen moment. Since no appointment is necessary, they come when it is most convenient, most practical (e.g., does not conflict with work scheduled, children not in school) or most meaningful (a key moment to deal with a life problem). Some arrive because they were passing by and saw the "no appointment necessary" sign. Some come because a critical episode has occurred with a longstanding issue (an employer threatens to fire a client when he once again arrives late for work). Some come to deal with an immediate crisis. Since clients arrive at their moment of choosing, they are likely to be highly motivated. Seeing clients at opportune moments is rewarding for therapists and promotes positive outcomes. At Our Lady of the Lake University's (OLLU) Community Counseling Service, about 50% of clients who schedule a first appointment do not show up. How many of those clients would have accessed counseling if they could just walk-in? We have no way of knowing, but we assume that some of them would.

- In Chapter Two, we summarize research that indicates that minority populations have a higher therapy dropout rate and are less likely to access traditional mental health services. In spite of remarkable increases in mental health services and providers, underserved populations still face obstacles to treatment: clients may not know how to initiate the process; social and cultural factors stigmatize mental illness; beliefs about healing may not include psychotherapy as a way to solve problems; the appointment-making process can be intimidating; long waiting lists for appointments; transportation; work schedules; and lack of child care. It is no wonder many in our community are discouraged about mental health services (Bobele et al., 2008). A walk-in counseling service can address many of these issues. Our walk-in service in San Antonio serves a high percentage of Latino clients, and it seems to a good fit. Clients can come at a time that fits into their schedule, they do not have to wait, and they do not need to commit to longer term services.

- A walk-in service is a way of dealing with a lengthy waiting list (Chapters Six and Eight). Certain hours of the week are set aside as walk-in times, and all clients requesting counseling services can be asked to walk-in as a way of getting started at the agency. Thus, the walk-in service can eliminate the need for a separate intake service. A certain percentage of walk-in clients (perhaps 50% or more) will be satisfied with their single walk-in session and not require further ongoing counseling by appointment. This will reduce the length of wait time for other agency counseling services. The agency will serve more clients more quickly with the same number on staff. The bottleneck at the point of entry will have eased or been erased.

- A walk-in service can be rewarding for therapists. Walk-in clients are motivated to have therapeutic conversations focused on change. There are no "no shows." Most walk-in services are organized so that sessions are about 50-minutes long, leaving time for therapists to complete a brief session note. (In Chapter Eight, Young describes a walk-in service in which the session note is completed as a part of the session itself with a copy given to the client as the session ends.) Once a walk-in session and session note are completed there is usually no more work to be done—no follow-up phone calls, no missed appointments to deal with. Only the administrative task of collecting from insurers and third party papers may remain. It is straightforward and the therapist, like the client, usually feels a sense of accomplishment.

- Walk-in counseling services can benefit mental health professionals and professionals in training. Two of the services described in this book, one in Calgary, Alberta, Canada and the other in Minneapolis, Minnesota (Chapters Five and Six) are operated in whole or in part by professionals who volunteer their time. Professionals volunteer because there is a learning environment created by the team approach and because they appreciate the chance to contribute to the well-being of their communities. The team format can also support graduate student training and those who require supervised experience for licensing. In a walk-in service, emerging professionals gain lots of experience in a short period of time. A wide variety of clientele access a walk-in service and the single-session nature of many of the cases means trainees have the opportunity to work with a large number of clients. Our graduate students at OLLU gain a great deal of confidence and experience through the walk-in aspect of our counseling center (Chapter Seven).

- Walk-in services serve as a safety valve for the community. After the walk-in service was operating in Calgary for about a year, a school counselor was asked for feedback about this new community resource. She said, "The Eastside Family Centre (EFC) is my savior." She explained that prior to the existence of EFC, she would recommend counseling for a child or family and would often receive feedback that the counseling services had a long wait list or that the fees were too high. At that point, some families were even more distressed. "Now," she said, "I can suggest EFC and tell them they can go that same day without an appointment and that there is no fee. It makes my job so much easier."

  A "no wait" service also means that clients can receive counseling while in the midst of a crisis. Clients have walked in the day after being sexually assaulted, shortly after a car accident, or after an episode of family violence. One father walked in with his 11-year-old daughter shortly after he had physically assaulted her. Her face showed bruising. He said, "I know I've blown it." Father and daughter were supported through the process of beginning to address their relationship issues and of contacting the child protection authorities. (In Chapter Ten we see how the principles of walk-in counseling were applied in assisting residents of Louisiana in the aftermath of Hurricane Katrina.)

- A walk-in service can be an important component of a larger network of mental health and social service resources (Chapters Six and Nine). Many who access a walk-in service have not had counseling before. They are searching for a resource that will address their needs. Through the walk-in service, they will learn about other community resources that are a good fit for their particular issues. Their walk-in session becomes a starting point for further services. Hospital emergency services send clients to walk-in services for a session of counseling after they have been assessed. Conversely, therapists at a walk-in clinic may send high risk clients to an emergency room for possible hospitalization or they put clients in touch with child protection services. A client whose therapist is on vacation may use a walk-in service for a booster session or to deal with an immediate crisis (Mallozzi, 2009).

Frequently Asked Questions about Walk-in Counseling

Don't some clients have problems that are too severe or too chronic for a single session walk-in service?

At a walk-in service, we don't choose our clients; they choose us. There is no pre-screening or assessment. The worst that can happen is that the client has a one-hour counseling session and is ultimately redirected to a more appropriate resource. But we also adhere to the principle that any client can benefit from a single session of therapy. For example, we do not treat schizophrenia. We can, however, assist people with serious mental health diagnoses to address their life problems. For example, a client diagnosed with schizophrenia was concerned that his landlord was going to evict him because he was talking to himself while in the halls of his apartment building. In addition to advising the client to consult with his psychiatrist about his medication, we role played how to have a reassuring conversation with the landlord. Another client with a longstanding history of depression wanted to use her walk-in session to discuss ideas that would help her get out of bed early enough to get to work on time.

Aren't there some clients who want something that a walk-in counseling session cannot give them?

Yes, that happens. In Chapter 3 you will learn that we want our clients to tell us as soon as possible what they want from the session. One reason for that is so that we can learn quickly if the client wants a service we cannot provide. For example, occasionally a client want a formal assessment or a professional letter of opinion. Another client might ask for medication or mistakenly believe that we offer ongoing counseling services by appointment. In each of those instances, we inform the client that we do not provide that service and offer information about where to get it. Sometimes after being so informed the client still wants their hour of counseling and we negotiate an achievable goal. Even when that does not occur, the session can still instill hope and optimism. We end every session with an assessment of the client's strengths.

What about clients who want to walk in again and again?

Actually, we routinely invite our walk-in clients to return. In that sense, walk-in counseling differs from single-session therapy. At the EFC more than 30% of clients have been there before. Sometimes they return after a few days or weeks and sometimes after several years. We are pleased when a client returns for another walk-in session. We think that means we're doing a good job.

In some important ways, though, a walk-in service is different from an ongoing counseling service. Similar to a walk-in medical clinic, clients who return may or may not see the same therapist. However, by reviewing previous session notes the new therapist will take into account what was done before. Unlike a traditional therapeutic relationship, we want our clients to develop a relationship to the service instead of the individual therapists. As a practical matter, the therapists in many walk-in clinics, especially volunteers and students, are not likely to be available when clients return. A very small percentage of clients choose to treat a walk-in service as if it is an ongoing psychotherapy service. Sometimes they can be accommodated, especially if repeat visits are not disruptive to the clinic. In other instances, clients are encouraged to connect with another, more appropriate, institution.

How can a walk-in service respond to at-risk clients?

A walk-in counseling service is more likely than most outpatient settings to attract clients dealing with immediate crises. So it is not surprising that some of our clients will present with issues of risk. Risks might include child abuse, elder abuse, domestic violence, threats of violence to others, and suicide or self-harm. (Chapter Five describes clients who use a walk-in counseling facility to disclose boundary crossing in relationships with professionals.) In each crisis, we work collaboratively with the client and significant others to assess the risk as well as the strengths and resources that can be incorporated in the development of a safety plan. When we are required to report to child protection authorities or the legal system, we do so. In those instances we make every effort to make the process as collaborative as possible with the client and significant others. For example, a family recently came to the CCS concerned that one of the young children had been sexually abused by a relative. We facilitated an on-the-spot phone call. The child's mother was advised that Child Protective Services (CPS) was the agency that could help her. She was relieved that we could assist her in this difficult procedure in a timely fashion.

In other situations, plans are made to assist a highly suicidal client in going to a hospital emergency room. That plan could involve a family member or, if necessary, the police accompanying the client to the emergency room. In some high risk situations, the usual 50-minute hour may go by the wayside. The session lasts as long as is necessary.

Can't a walk-in service be overwhelmed with more clients than it can handle?

"You'll be overwhelmed" was a comment we sometimes heard in the months preceding the opening of the EFC. Because our desire was to address the issue of accessibility of mental health services, we took this worry as a sign that we must be on the right track—we really were about to make services more available to our community. Of course, we didn't know how many people would come. When we first opened our doors, after a promotional effort in the community, utilization was low. Gradually, though, business increased. (In subsequent chapters you will see information about utilization rates in various walk-in services.) While this happens infrequently, we've found that occasionally more clients walk in than can be handled on a given shift. When that occurs we do some triaging. The supervisor/shift coordinator and the reception/intake person review waiting clients' intake forms to ensure that any clients who might be at risk get a session. Those not seen are told that they will be "put at the head of the line" if they return.

Isn't this a superficial, band-aid approach?

We've been asked this question so many times that we decided to do some Google research on the topic of bandages (Wikipedia). According to archaeologists, bandages have been around at least since the time the pyramids were being built in Egypt. They are a long-term hit that transcends geography and culture. Recently, public health researchers have suggested that, if anything, we do not use bandages enough. They recommend that for many injuries, bandages could be used more frequently and for a longer time period. The reasons for the centuries long utilization of this relatively low tech invention are simple: Bandages promote healing and prevent the spread of infection. So when we're asked if walk-in counseling is a band-aid approach we say, "Yes. Thank you for the compliment."

Is walk-in counseling primarily for low-income and minority groups?

The walk-in services described in this book serve a high percentage of low-income clients. This is due to the cost efficiency of a walk-in service for both clients and funders and to the fact that walking in is a logical choice for those who have difficulty planning ahead or are in immediate crises (circumstances that many low-income people face on a daily basis). A significant percentage of walk-in clients are from minority cultural and ethnic groups. Walk-in services are culturally syntonic for some minorities that are very familiar with walk-in medical clinics, emergency rooms, and church confessionals. However, we urge the reader not to assume that single, walk-in sessions are designed only for low income and minority clients. Many clients are Caucasian and some are well off financially. Whether a walk-in single session is a good fit depends on the person and the context; it is not an issue of whether walking is a better or a lesser service.

Why Not Walk-in Therapy?

We think there are good reasons for therapists and agencies to carefully consider whether they want to add the option of walking in to their compliment of services. For therapists, walk-in sessions are not for the faint of heart. An outcome is required in just an hour. This can challenge the mindset and clinical strategies for many therapists. (While Chapter 3 proposes a framework that can reduce stress for the walk-in therapist, walk-in work still requires that therapists and clients collaborate to produce a positive outcome in an hour.) An agency may discover that some of their therapists are disinclined to take that leap. The agency will also have to consider that a walk-in service is likely to have an impact on other programs. For example, what will it mean for the waiting list and the intake coordinator role? Some walk-in clients will decide that their single session is sufficient for now and will not be referred to other agency programs. The average length of treatment may drop in other counseling services that the agency operates. While this creates the potential for the agency to serve more clients with a similar number of staff, it can be a big adjustment. Planning is essential and buy in by the professional staff is a crucial element.

What Follows

This is the first book that comprehensively addresses the topic of walk-in, single-session therapy. It proposes a new paradigm of clinical service delivery that is designed to meet the changing demands of the 21st century. As mental health resources diminish, they become less and less available to many of those who are most in need. The U.S. Surgeon General reports that only half of those who would benefit from treatment seek help.

One finding of the Surgeon General's report is that the complex and fragmented mental health service delivery system in the United States, financial barriers, and social stigma all help create barriers to a full range of services. The report proposes that the mental health field is plagued with more barriers to service than any other area of health and medicine. (Miller & Slive, 2004, p. 95).

Wait lists are growing and 50% of those who wait for appointments do not show up (Barrett, Chua, Crits-Christoph, & Gibbons, 2008). Traditionally, public mental health outpatient services require that clients wait for an intake session that is often followed by a further wait period. We are proposing a form of service delivery that could eliminate the wait for those mental health services. It provides an immediate entry point to services and relieves some of the anguish of clients and referral sources by providing hassle-free access, at times determined by client need. It makes use of pragmatic, solution-oriented approaches that focus on practical goals that are most relevant to the client.

This is a practical book that can be used by practitioners, educators, and mental health program planners. It shows how walk-in therapy can play a significant role in a service delivery system. It reviews research about the frequency and efficacy of brief therapy and single sessions (Chapter Two). It provides ideas about how to effectively conduct single sessions (Chapter Three). It also describes how walk-in services have been implemented in a variety of clinical contexts in Canada and the United States. These contexts are:

- A counseling center that serves all ages and in which walk-in counseling is its centerpiece (Chapter Six);
- An agency that focuses on children and families and developed a walk-in service to replace its traditional intake service, thereby serving more clients and decreasing its wait list (Chapter Eight);
- The impact of a center in which professionals have volunteered to provide walk-in sessions for more than forty years (Chapter Five);
- A walk-in counseling service that is a component of large coordinated health and mental health service delivery system (Chapter Nine);
- The application of walk-in counseling concepts to survivors of Hurricane Katrina (Chapter Ten);
- Walk-in counseling as a component of the training of graduate students in a university-sponsored, community-based counseling service (Chapter Seven);

Numerous case examples are provided. They include individuals, couples and families, clients of all ages, and a wide variety of presenting concerns that range from immediate crises to longstanding diagnostic conditions. The clients are Canadian and American, Latino/Latina, African American, aboriginal, and Caucasian. Our intent is to give the reader a broad overview of the current state of walk-in single-session counseling and specific ideas about how to conduct these sessions.

A note should also be made here about our Index. As both the theory and practice of walk-in, single-session therapy continue to evolve, many definitions and practices are anecdotal and change with the circumstance and location of the practice. We've designed the Index to reflect this vibrant state by listing key words both by concept and by location, as they are brought to life in the six clinics described in this book.

References

Barrett, M. S., Chua, W., Crits-Christoph, P., Gibbons, M., & Thompson, D. (2008). Early withdrawal from mental health treatment: Implications for psychotherapy practice. *Psychotherapy: Theory, Research, Practice, Training,* 45, 247-267.

Bobele, M., Lopez, S..-G., Scamardo, M., & Solórzano, B. (2008). Single-

Session walk-in therapy with Mexican-American clients. *Journal of Systemic Therapies,* 27(4), 75-89.

Hoyt, M. (2009). *Brief Psychotherapies: Principles & Practice.* Phoenix, AZ: Zeig, Tucker & Theisen.

Mallozzi, V. Answers to life's worries, in 3 minute bursts. *The New York Times.* August, 30, 2009.

Miller, J. & Slive, A. (2004). Breaking down the barriers to clinical service delivery: Walk-in family therapy. *Journal of Marital and Family Therapy, 30*, 95-103.

Talmon, M. (1990). *Single-session therapy.* San Francisco: Jossey-Bass.

Chapter 2

The Research Case for Walk-In Single Sessions

Kyle Green, MS, Teresa Correia, MS, Monte Bobele, Ph.D. and *Arnie Slive, Ph.D.*

This chapter will provide an overview of the research in extremely brief therapy in general, single-session therapy in particular and walk-in therapies. A recent review of a half-century's research on psychotherapy outcomes concluded that time-limited and time-unlimited therapies are comparably effective (Orlinsky, Rùnnestad, & Willutzki, 2004). In fact, the topic of brief therapy used to occupy a unique section of Bergin and Garfield's authoritative handbooks of psychotherapy and behavior change. Shapiro et al (2003) point out that the most recent edition (Lambert, 2004) no longer makes such a distinction and conclude that brief therapies (25 sessions or less) have become the standard. Moreover, a new distinction is being proposed—ultra brief therapy (six or fewer sessions). Clearly, a confluence of economic, public-policy, theoretical, and other pragmatic factors are contributing to a rethinking of how much therapy is sufficient. Walk-in and single-session therapies (SST) are firmly entrenched at the briefest end of these ultra-brief therapies.

Related areas of research, pertinent to the current work on single-session therapy, are the dose-response literature and the phase models of psychotherapy outcomes (Baldwin, Berkeljon, Atkins, Olsen, & Nielsen 2009; Feaster, Newman, & Rice, 2003; Hansen, 2003; Harnett, O'Donovan, & Lambert, 2010; Lambert & Forman, 2003; Wolgast, et. al., 2003). These models, based on meta-analyses of outcome studies describe substantial improvements in the early stages of psychotherapy followed by ever-decreasing improvements as psychotherapy continues. Graphs of this phenomenon typically show a steep rise in improvement in the first through eighth sessions of therapy, with improvement approaching an asymptote beyond the eighth session.

Commonly, clients make dramatic improvements during the beginning of a therapy experience and that improvement declines as the number of therapy sessions increases (Bloom, 2001; Howard, Kopta, Krause, & Orlinsky, 1986; Seligman, 1995). This suggests that it may be a myth that therapy has to be lengthy to be effective (Silverman & Beech, 1984). Askevold (1983), for example, found that there were no outcome differences between three randomly assigned treatment groups: single-session therapy, brief therapy, and traditional therapy of women with anorexia nervosa.

Who Uses Walk-in Services?

Several walk-in services have addressed the question of who uses their services. At the Community Counseling Service (CCS), in San Antonio, the clients who use our walk-in service are very similar to the overall demographics in our clinic (Chapter Seven). The clinic serves a largely Hispanic population, particularly Mexican-Americans. Most have incomes below $20,000. The presenting issues range from school-related issues to life-threatening crises. Karen Young (Chapter 8) highlights the types of concerns that most often bring clients to seek out walk-in services at the Reach Out Centre for Kids (ROCK) in Ontario, Canada. Most often the clients report problems related to anxiety, depression, relationships, and anger. On average, clients endured these problems for a year before they access services at the clinic. She also explores reasons clients gave for using the walk-in service. She finds that the recommendation of others, immediate accessibility, and the need for additional services were most prevalent. Harper-Jaques and Leahy (Chapter Nine) have also kept track of the types of problems clients reported in South Calgary as reasons for attending their walk-in service. The authors report depression, anxiety, and relationship concerns as most prevalent. They further add that very few clients who utilize the walk-in service require a higher level of care. Gary Shoener (Chapter Five) also provides a detailed description of the types of clients seen at his walk-in counseling service in Minneapolis. He reports that

41% have family incomes less than $10,000 a year, and that about half of the service's clients have no insurance coverage. Furthermore, of those clients who have insurance, many are burdened with high co-pays or large deductibles, limited access to providers, and long wait times for an appointment.

Are Walk-in Clients Satisfied with Services?

Whether or not clients received the help that they had hoped for is an important consideration in evaluating walk-in services. Although researchers and clinicians frequently establish outcome measures based on their theories or third party standards, we think that clients' evaluations of our services are important.

A number of studies have directly investigated clients' satisfaction with their experience in a walk-in clinic. In an early study Silverman and Beech (1984) explored the relationship between the length of therapy and client-assessed outcomes. The authors found that clients' satisfaction ratings of both unplanned single-sessions and multi-sessions are highly similar and remarkably favorable. The majority of clients in both groups reported that the interventions had been helpful. Nearly 80% of the participants in both the single-session and multi-session groups reported that the problem for which they had sought assistance had been solved. The authors also noted that while therapists' perceptions of client improvement were related to duration of the intervention, the clients' perceptions were not.

More recently, outcomes and client satisfaction have been extensively researched in several studies at the Eastside Family Center (EFC) in Calgary. Miller and Slive (2004) contacted 43 clients after a walk-in session to assess satisfaction with services and clinical improvement. The majority of respondents were satisfied with the services and 68% reported improvement. Lawson, Miller, and Slive (2006) contacted 100 clients who attended walk-in single-session therapy and the majority expressed satisfaction with the model and the services received. Miller (2008) surveyed 403 of Calgary's EFC walk-in clients. Like Silverman and Beech, Miller's participants reported favorable experiences with a single-session of walk-in therapy. Of the former clients surveyed, over 80% reported they were "very satisfied," or "satisfied," with the single-session therapy approach. Remarkably, less than 2% reported being dissatisfied. Like the Silverman and Beech study, this article provides rationale for continuing research on SST, particularly on how it impacts, and can potentially benefit, mental health consumers. Clements, McElheran, Hackney, and Park (Chapter Six) asked 50 previous walk-in service recipients at the EFC to complete a follow-up survey. Those who completed the survey (90%) reported that they were satisfied with the overall walk-in therapy experience. The EFC estimates approximately 2200 clients attend walk-in sessions per year. Clients are administered a Session Rating Scale (SRS) (Duncan, Miller, & Reynolds, et al, 2003) at the end of every session to determine therapy success and to evaluate the client/therapist relationship. Clements and his colleagues (Chapter 6) analyzed five years worth of SRS data and determined that clients rated 85-90% agreement with the four positive statements (Relationship, Goals and Topics, Approach or Method, and Overall) of the SRS, reflecting a strong therapeutic alliance was developed.

In another study of a walk-in clinic in Calgary, Syverson (2006) reviewed 188 walk-in cases seen at the Mental Health Walk-In at South Calgary Health Center (MHWI) and found that 80% of their clients were satisfied with the knowledge and caring nature of the staff. Syverson also reported that clients' pre-session distress level was significantly reduced by the end of the session. Young (Chapter 8) also discusses satisfaction at The Reach Out Center for Kids (ROCK) in Ontario, Canada, which provides walk-in services to approximately 1500 families per year. Approximately 50% attend only one session of therapy (i.e., these are clients who do not return after their walk-in session or do not schedule appointment for further service). Each family is given an evaluation survey at the end of each session. Young examined the 2008-2009 evaluations that were returned to the clinic (50%) and found that 89% of clients felt the session assisted them with the problem that brought them to therapy and 92% reported that they would return to the ROCK if they needed to in the future. Harper-Jaques & Leahy (Chapter 9) further describe positive results in their evaluation of client pre- and post- levels of distress and satisfaction of services at their MHWI Program located in the South Calgary Health Centre (SCHC). The findings consistently showed that clients who received walk-in services at MHWI experienced a significant decrease in distress levels. In summary, it appears clients are indeed satisfied with walk-in services and report positive outcomes.

Have Single-Session and Walk-in Therapies Been Effective?

Now we want to examine the effectiveness of single-session and walk-in therapies. We have known for some time that the most frequent, or modal, number of therapy sessions is one (Boyhan, 1996; Bloom, 1992; Talmon, 1990). Baekeland & Lundwall (1975) found that 20% -57% of general psychiatric patients did not return after their initial visit. Hoyt, Rosenbaum, and Talmon (1992) found that between 30% and 55% of clients are likely to attend only one therapy session. In government-run health services in the state of Victoria, Australia, over a three-year period, 42% of 115,00 clients attended only one session of therapy, even though clients were routinely invited to return (J. Young, personal communication, January 24, 2009). We will look at single-session and walk-in therapies in turn.

For the most part, walk-in clinics operate on a single-session therapy model. However, not all single-session therapy is conducted in walk-in clinics. Some single sessions are scheduled by appointment. First we will review the evidence that single-session therapies are effective, and then we will turn to the research unique to walk-in clinics.

Single-Session Therapies

Talmon described the three logical classifications of single-session therapy: planned, unplanned and those that result from a mutual decision by the therapist and client that no more sessions are needed. Planned single-session therapy occurs in and out of walk-in clinics. Some clinics provide a single consultation appointment that clients and therapist understand will be the only appointment. The therapist plans to meet only once with a client and the client is aware of this arrangement. The second type occurs when, at the end of the initial consultation, the therapist and client agree that the client's goals have been met and future sessions are not necessary. Finally, and perhaps least understood, are the times when clients fail to return for a scheduled appointment after the first session. In these instances, therapists plan subsequent sessions, clients schedule another session, and clients either do not appear for the scheduled appointment or call to cancel additional treatment. This third category of single-session therapy is referred to by various terms such as premature termination, drop out, and treatment failure.

Research on planned single-session therapy

In his 1990 book, Talmon and his colleagues documented that clients reported improvement after one session of therapy. Talmon and his colleagues contacted 58 former clients with various presenting concerns who had received a planned single-session of therapy for a follow-up interview three to twelve months later. Of those, 88% reported "much improvement" or "improvement" following the session and 79% stated that one session was sufficient to address their presenting concerns. Only three clients reported that one session had not been sufficient to address their concerns. In an attempt to replicate Talmon's findings, Kaffman (1995) reviewed the charts of 211 clients' charts who had received services over a three-year period. These clients were contacted up to six years after their initial session. Kaffman reported that 64 (30%) of the 211 clients said they had met their goals for therapy in one session. Of these 64, 84% had mutually agreed to end therapy after one session. In another early study, Baer, Marlatt, Kivlahan, Fromme, and Larimer (1992) studied three approaches to therapy with teen clients in an alcohol risk reduction class. Each group of teens was randomly assigned to a six-week class, a six-unit self study manual, or a single one-hour feedback session. Comparable outcome results were reported across groups initially and after a two-year follow-up period. This suggests that a single-session of therapy was as effective as lengthier and more expensive interventions.

More recent brief therapy research has found between 50-70% of clients showed positive improvement after attending one or two sessions (Barkham et al., 2006; Cahill et al., 2003). In his meta-analysis, Bloom (2001) found that one single interview could be as effective as long-term psychotherapy. According to Bloom, the outcomes of planned short-term psychotherapy and time-unlimited psychotherapy were generally the same (Bloom, 1997).

Oest (1989) found that 18 of 20 women who attended a 2-hour single-session of therapy for specific phobias showed improvement or completely recovered following the session. Lokshin, Lindgren, Weinberger, and Koviach (1991) conducted single sessions of therapy with nine children who had habitual coughs not associated with asthma or other physiological findings. Seven of the children were contacted two years later; six were symptom free. Meanwhile, Campbell (1999) reviewed outcomes of 44 clients who were seen for a single-session of therapy in a family service agency. Seventy-five percent reported significant improvement six weeks following the appointment. Coverly, Garralda, and Bowman (1995) looked at the long-term effects of a single-session, standardized psychiatric intervention in primary care for mothers of children with psychiatric disorders. Of the 14 mothers who returned follow-up questionnaires, nine reported that the intervention had been markedly or extremely useful. All nine of these mothers also indicated that being able to talk about their problems and the specific advice given to them had been helpful, while seven of these mothers showed appreciation for having been able to talk to someone who understood them and gave them reassurance. Three mothers noted that it had been useful to receive a better understanding of their problems. This study again demonstrates the helpfulness of SST in working with families systems and presents specific feedback from participants on some qualities that contributed to its success.

In a recent study with families, Sommers-Flanagan (2007) noted that parents had very positive reactions to a planned single-session consultation experience and rated themselves as less stressed and more capable of handling their children's difficult behavior as a result. Goodman and Happell (2006) found that 56 out of 90 families surveyed reported that their problems were much or a little better following a single-session consultation. Of these 90 families, 70 reported that the consultation had been very helpful or somewhat helpful.

Perkins and her team (2006) implemented single-session, 2-hour semi-structured assessments and treatment interventions for children, their caregivers, and household siblings. Approaching each session as if it were to be the only one, the team used a solution-focused family therapy approach. Perkins' findings demonstrated that those families who received a single-session of therapy showed clinically significant improvement over a control group that was put on a waiting list for six weeks. Furthermore, the level of clients' satisfaction with therapy was also high, with many parents indicating that they preferred the rapid treatment. In a follow-up, Perkins and Scarlett (2008) conducted an 18-month follow up with participants from the 2006 study. Using identical measures to evaluate the long-term effectiveness of SST, they found no significant differences in the clients' presenting problems, severity of the clients' presenting problems, psychopathology, or client satisfaction. They also found that 60% of the original study's clients maintained significant improvement following their one session of therapy, while the remaining 40% benefited from additional sessions of SST. However, those who attended only one session of SST, and did not require additional sessions, had greater improvement in ratings of problem severity. Perkins and Scarlett concluded that SST can be "an efficient and effective first form of treatment" for children and adolescents with mental health needs (p. 154).

Research on Unplanned Single-session Therapy

Hoyt (2009) noted that it is common for psychotherapists to view a client ending therapy as "early withdrawal." But there is more and more evidence suggesting that clients are satisfied with the results of one session and do not need to return. As an example of researchers who focused on the "problem" of few sessions, Pekarik (1992a) reported that problem resolution, extraneous variables preventing access to treatment, and treatment dissatisfaction were the three most prevalent reasons clients gave for terminating treatment. Barrett, Chua, Crits-Cristoph, Gibbons, and Thompson (2008) similarly identified reasons why clients only attended one session of therapy, which included resistance, lack of motivation, external barriers to treatment, and client expectations regarding the length of treatment. The authors then described implications resulting from early termination such as significant financial burden on mental health agencies, lower morale amongst mental health clinicians, and diminished access for others in need.

The following studies explored the relationship between length of therapy, outcomes, and client satisfaction. Pekarik (1992b) found increased Brief Symptom Inventory (BSI) symptom improvement in "problem improved" dropouts when compared to ongoing clients, which highlighted a discrepancy between therapists' and clients' reports of symptom improvement within the dropout group. He also found that the therapists in his study perceived all drop-outs as being unimproved.

Other reasons for early termination have also been reported. For example, Battino (2007) reviewed research conducted by brief therapists at the Brief Family Therapy Center (BFTC) in Milwaukee, Wisconsin. In the research, the clinic receptionist told clients prior to beginning their first session that they would receive either five or ten sessions. The purpose of the study was to look at how client expectations for therapy length could affect the actual length of therapy. It is not clear how the number of sessions was identified, but the therapists were not informed of the client's expectation of the number of sessions that they would receive. Once therapy was terminated and the clients' charts were reviewed, it was discovered that client's began doing "significant therapeutic work" about one or two sessions prior to their expected final session. The only difference between the two treatment groups was the client's expectation. This research speaks to how a client's expectation for therapy directly influences its length or duration.

Walk-in Therapies

Walk-In Research

There is a growing body of research describing the outcomes of walk-in treatment as it has being conducted in various centers throughout the United States and Canada. Several of the walk-in centers are described in this volume. Young (Chapter Eight) compared presession and postsession evaluations completed by 408 clients in Ontario who attended the Reach Out Centre for Kids (ROCK) walk-in services in a single year. The postsession evaluations showed that clients reported that they thought they had more coping strategies and increased confidence to solve their own problems as a result of the single session of therapy that they had just completed. In order to evaluate the longer term effect of the walk-in single sessions a two-month follow-up questionnaire was completed by 100 of the study's original clients. Twenty-six clients reported their presenting issues remained resolved. Seventy-four clients reported their original presenting problem was still a concern but that they were significantly less worried, were more knowledgeable about community resources, and had more ideas about how to manage the problem. In a similar study at Calgary's Eastside Family Center (EFC), Clements, McElheran, Hackney, and Park (Chapter Six) analyzed five years' of clients' postsession rating scales. They reported that clients typically showed a 20-25% decrease in distress after their first therapy session. Taken together, these two studies suggest that a single-session of walk-in therapy can be helpful in reducing the stress present at the time of the initial appointment, and that the benefits of the session remain for some time afterwards.

Young (Chapter Eight) delved deeper into her former clients' evaluations of their walk-in session. She was particularly interested in what clients would report had been helpful about their session. She asked them to complete an open-ended questionnaire asking what they had learned during each session. Eight different themes emerged from the data: 1) increased self-awareness, 2) awareness of the impact of the problem, 3) increased awareness of resources, 4) more general knowledge about the nature of problem, 5) more knowledge of general strategies to help deal with the problem, 6) knowledge of specific techniques to manage mental health issues, 7) better communication skills, and 8) knowledge that children were willing to get help. These themes suggest that clients identified profound changes in their lives that resulted from their session. This might be surprising to critics of short-term therapies who fear that such therapies only address superficial issues in clients' lives.

Rates of clients returning for further sessions

Clements, McElheran, Hackney, and Park (Chapter Six) stated that 30-35% of clients return for another session within a one year period. That means that 65-70% of clients seen at the EFC attended only one session within a one year timeframe. Schoener (Chapter Five) further reported that the 1,588 clients seen in 2009 at a walk-in counseling service had attended 5,231 counseling sessions. A similar return rate was found at the Mental Health Walk-In Program. As Harper-Jaques & Leahey (Chapter Nine) point out, 31% of the clients seen during the 2009-2010 fiscal year had attended a single-session of therapy previously.

Economics of Employing Walk-in Services and Time-Limited Therapies

Managing waiting lists, cancelled appointments, no-shows, and other client scheduling issues can be a source of frustration for private practitioners and mental health clinics. Little research is available on the economic impact of failed appointments in mental health clinics, but family practice physicians have begun to analyze the effect in their practices. Moore et al (2001) examined the effect of no-shows, or missed appointments, at a family practice residency clinic. They reported average frequencies of no-show missed appointments (not including cancellations) across family practice centers between 6% and 26.1%, with some centers reporting rates as high as 50%. The researchers found that by incorporating a walk-in system to their regular scheduled appointments, they were able to recoup up to 89.5% of what would have been lost revenue from their no-show and cancelled appointments. In our experiences at the CCS (Chapter Seven), we found that walk-in clients frequently turn a therapist's idle hour into a productive one when a scheduled client fails to show up for an appointment.

Conclusion

In this chapter we have presented a broad overview of the research base for walk-in single-session therapy. Talmon (1990) recognized that SST might not be helpful for all clients. Clients who had found single-session therapy to be insufficient in dealing with their presenting problems sought a more traditional type of therapy, required inpatient hospitalization, were dealing with conditions believed to have strong biological or chemical components or clear neurological damage, or exhibited behaviors associated with a personality disorders diagnosis (Talmon 1990). Boyhan (1996) suggested that SST might not be sufficient to meet the needs of clients who were court mandated or referred by a protective agency. She also pointed out that clients who were being seen for problems related to sexual abuse, substance abuse, acquired brain injury, serious mental illness, HIV/AIDS, etc. might be better served by counselors who specialize in these areas. Bloom's (2001) meta-analysis found that SST is effective in treatment of the following areas: "intrapsychic difficulties, interpersonal conflict, and as an adjunct treatment for medical disorders" (p.75).

Miller and Slive (2004) suggested that access to a walk-in, SST service offered clients a valuable entry point into clinical services for occasions when longer-term outpatient therapy or other services is warranted. It also gave clients a chance to try out therapy and get a sense of what it can be like. Boyhan (1996) further highlighted that being able to quickly access SST, even when additional sessions are recommended, assists with reducing wait time for initial entry into treatment, can stabilize an immediate crisis, and increases client satisfaction toward mental health service providers or agencies. For these clients, it may also be helpful to think of single-session and walk-in services as forms of intermittent therapy in which there could be a number of single sessions over weeks, months or years.

We have shown that walk-in and planned single sessions are effective for children, adolescents and adults, produce high rates of client satisfaction, and have long lasting results. We need further research into: which clients would benefit most and least, training therapists in SST and the impact of walk-in services on mental health service networks and on communities.

References

Asay, T. P., Lambert, M. J., Gregersen, A. T., & Goates, M. K. (2002). Using patient-refocused research in evaluating treatment outcome in private practice. *Journal of Clinical Psychology, 58* (10), 1213-1225. doi: 10.1002/jclp.10107

Askevold, F. (1983). What are the helpful factors in psychotherapy for anorexia nervosa? *International Journal of Eating Disorders, 2,* 193-197.

Baekeland, F., & Lundwall. L. (1975) Dropping out of treatment: A critical review. *Psychological Bulletin, 82,* 738-783.

Baer, J. S., Marlatt, G. A., Kivlahan, D. R., Fromme, K., Larimer, M. E., & Williams, E. (1992). An experimental test of three methods of alcohol risk reduction with young adults. *Journal of Consulting Psychology, 60,* 974-979.

Baldwin, S. A., Berkeljon, A., Atkins, D. C., Olsen, J. A., & Nielsen, S. L. (2009). Rates of change in naturalistic psychotherapy: Contrasting dose-effect and good-enough level models of change. *Journal of Consulting & Clinical Psychology, 77,* 203-211. doi: 10.1037/a0015235

Barkham, M., Connell, J., Stiles, W., Miles, J., Margison, F., Evans, C., & Mellor-Clark, J. (2006). Dose-effect relations and responsive regulation of treatment duration: The good enough level. *Journal of Consulting and Clinical Psychology, 74* (1), 160.

Barrett, M. S., Chua, W. J., Crits-Cristoph, P., Gibbons, M. B., & Thompson, D. (2008). Early withdrawal from mental health treatment: Implications for psychotherapy practice. *Psychotherapy: Theory, Research, Practice, Training. 45,* 247-267.

Battino, R. (2007). Expectation: Principles and practice of very brief therapy. *Contemporary Hypnosis, 24*(1), 19-29.

Bloom, B. L. (1992). Planned short-term psychotherapy: A clinical handbook. Boston: Allen & Bacon.

Bloom, B. L. (1997). Planned short-term psychotherapy: A clinical handbook (2nd. Ed). Boston: Allyn and Bacon.

Bloom, B. L. (2001). Focused single-session psychotherapy: A review of the clinical and research literature. *Brief Treatment and Crisis Intervention, 1,* 75-86.

Boyhan, P. A. (1996). Client's perceptions of single-session consultations as an option to waiting for family therapy. *Australian and New Zealand Journal of Family Therapy, 17(2),* 85-96.

Cahill, J., Barkham, M., Hardy, G., Reese, A., Shapiro, D. A., Stiles, W. B., & Macaskill, N. (2003). Outcomes of patients completing and not completing cognitive therapy for depression. *British Journal of Clinical Psychology, 42,* 133-143.

Campbell, A. (1999). Single-session interventions: An example of clinical research in practice. *Australian and New Zealand Journal of Family Therapy, 20,* 183-194.

Coverly, C. T., Garralda, M. E., & Bowman, F. (1995). Psychiatric interventions in primary care for mothers whose school children have psychiatric disorder. *British Journal of General Practice, 45,* 235-237.

Duncan, B., Miller, D. S., Sparks, J. A., Claud, D. A., Reynolds, L. R., Brown, J., et al. (2003). The session rating scale: Preliminary psychometric properties of a "working" alliance measure. *Journal of Brief Therapy, 3*(1), 3-12.

Feaster, D. J., Newman, F. L., & Rice, C. (2003). Longitudinal analysis when the experimenter does not determine when treatment ends: what is dose, response? [Article]. *Clinical Psychology & Psychotherapy, 10* (6), 352-360. doi: 10.1002/cpp.382

Goodman, D., & Happell, B. (2006). The efficacy of family intervention in adolescent health. *The International Journal of Psychiatric Nursing Research, 12,* 1364-1377.

Hansen, N. B., & Lambert, M. J. (2003). An evaluation of the dose-response relationship in naturalistic treatment settings using survival analysis. *Mental Health Services Research, 5*(1), 1-12. doi: 10.1023/a:1021751307358

Harnett, P., O'Donovan, A., & Lambert, M. J. (2010). The dose response relationship in psychotherapy: Implications for social policy. *Clinical Psychologist, 14,* 39-44. doi: 10.1080/13284207.2010.500309

Howard, K. I., Kopta, S. M., Krause, M. S., & Orlinsky, D. E. (1986). The dose-effect relationship in psychotherapy. *American Psychologist, 41,* 159-164.

Hoyt, M. F. (1984). Single-session solutions. In M. F. Hoyt (Ed.), *Constructive therapies* (pp. 140-159). New York, NY: Guilford Press.

Hoyt, M. F. (2009). *Brief psychotherapies: Principles and practices.* Phoenix, AZ: Zeig, Tucker, & Thiesen, Inc.

Hoyt, M., Rosenbaum, R., & Talmon, M. (1992). Planned single-session therapy. In S. H. Budman, M. Hoyt, & S. Friedman (Eds.), The first session in brief therapy. New York: Guilford Press.

Kaffman, M. (1995). Brief therapy in the Israeli Kibbutz. *Contemporary Family Therapy, 17,* 449-468.

Lambert, M. J. (2004). Bergin and Garfield's handbook of psychotherapy and behavior change (5th ed.). New York, NY: Wiley.

Lambert, M., & Forman, E. (2002). The psychotherapy dose-response effect and its implications for treatment delivery services. *Clinical Psychology: Science and Practice, 9* (3), 330.

Lawson, A., McElheran, N., & Slive, A. (1997). Single-session walk-in therapy: A model for the 21st century. *Family Therapy News, 30* (4), 15–25.

Lokshin, B., Lindgren, S., Weinberger, J., & Koviach, J. (1991). Outcome of habit cough in children with a brief session of suggestion therapy. *Annals of Allergy, 67,* 579-582.

Miller, J. K. (2008). Walk-in single-session team therapy: A study of client satisfaction. *Journal of Systemic Therapies, 27(3),* 78-94.

Miller, J. K. & Slive, A. (2004). Breaking down the barriers to clinical service delivery: Walk-in family therapy. *Journal of Marital and Family Therapy, 30,* 95-105.

Moore, C., P. Wilson-Witherspoon, et al. (2001). Time and money: effects of no-shows at a family practice residency clinic. *Family Medicine-Kansas City.* 33(7): 522-527.

Oest, L. G. (1989). One-session treatment for specific phobias. *Behavior Research and Therapy, 7,* 1-7.

Orlinsky, D. E., Rùnnestad, M. H., & Willutzki, U. (2004). Fifty years of psychotherapy process-outcome research: Continuity and change. In M. J. Lambert (Ed.), *Bergin and Garfeld's Handbook of Psychotherapy and Behaviour Change.* New York: Wiley.

Pekarik, G. (1992a). Relationship of clients' reasons for dropping out of treatment to outcome and satisfaction. *Journal of Clinical Psychology, 48,* 91-98.

Pekarik, G. (1992b). Posttreatment adjustment of clients who drop out early vs. late in treatment. *Journal of Clinical Psychology, 48,* 379-387.

Perkins, R. (2006). The effectiveness of one session of therapy using a single-session therapy approach for children and adolescents with mental health problems. Psychology, Psychotherapy, 79(Pt 2), 215-227. doi: 10.1348/147608305X60523

Perkins, R., & Scarlett, G. (2008). The effectiveness of single-session therapy in child and adolescent mental health. Part 2: An 18-month follow-up study. *Psychology & Psychotherapy: Theory, Research & Practice, 81(2),* 143-156.

Seligman, M. E. P. (1995). The effectiveness of psychotherapy: The *Consumer Reports* study. *American Psychologist, 50,* 965-974. doi: 10.1037/0003-066x.50.12.965

Shapiro, D. A., Barkham, M., Stiles, W. B., Hardy, G. E., Rees, A., Reynolds, S., & Startup, M. (2003). Time is of the essence: A selective review of the fall and rise of brief therapy research. *Psychology & Psychotherapy: Theory, Research & Practice, 76,* 211-235.

Silverman, W. H., & Beech, R. P. (1984). Length of intervention and client assessed outcome. *Journal of Clinical Psychology, 40,* 475-480.

Sommers-Flanagan, J. (2007). Single-session consultations for parents: A preliminary investigation. *The Family Journal: Counseling and Therapy for Couples and Families, 15,* 24-29.

Syverson, A. (2006). South Calgary Health Centre new mental health service evaluation. Calgary, Alberta Canada: Calgary Health Region.

Talmon, M. (1990). Single-session therapy: Maximizing the effect of the first (and often only) therapeutic encounter. San Francisco: Jossey-Bass Publishers.

Wolgast, B. M., Lambert, M. J., & Puschner, B. (2003). The Dose-Response Relationship at a College Counseling Center: Implications for Setting Session Limits. *Journal of College Student Psychotherapy, 18* (2), 15-29. doi: 10.1300/J035v18n02.

Chapter 3

Making a Difference in 50 Minutes: A Framework for Walk-in Counselling

Arnie Slive, Ph.D. and *Monte Bobele, Ph.D.*

We have provided walk-in counseling for approximately 20 years in a variety of settings in Canada and the United States (Bobele, Lopez, Scamardo & Solórzano, 2008; Slive, McElheran, & Lawson, 2008; Slive, McElheran, & Lawson, 2001; Slive, MacLalurin, Oakander, & Amundson, 1995). The settings are both rural and urban; the clients include children, adults, and families with wide ranging presenting concerns. Our work has involved direct service as well as supervision and training. Based on this experience, we have developed a framework that serves to guide us in our walk-in work. This framework is not based on a particular model of therapy, though postmodern, social constructivist, and family systems approaches have been major influences. In fact, we believe that many models of psychotherapy can be readily adapted to this framework. The purpose of this chapter is to describe our framework for conducting walk-in sessions. We begin with a description of a mindset, or set of beliefs, that support the notion that many clients want therapy to be as brief as possible and that significant change can occur rapidly. This is followed by a description of the context in which we do our walk-in work. We then describe the underlying tenets of our work and the "how to's" of the practice framework. The chapter concludes with a detailed case example.

A Single-Session Mindset

A therapist's own belief in the effectiveness of brief therapy is a crucial element in conducting successful walk-in sessions. We encourage our trainees to familiarize themselves with the research about length of therapy (Chapter Two) emphasizing:

- the frequency with which single-sessions occur in all models of therapy,
- the fact that change occurs early in the course of therapy, and
- the effectiveness of single-session and brief therapy.

Jay Haley said to a student preparing for a first session with a client: "Maybe you don't have a case really, except for the first interview. That would be nice I think. Every therapist should shoot for one session (Haley & Richeport-Haley, 2003 p.33)."

Consistent with Haley, in our training of graduate students we have developed a motto:

Every Case Has The Potential To Be A Single-Session Case!

This motto, like a mantra, is repeated continuously throughout the training period. It serves to keep our students focused on the idea that this first session may be the only one. Walk-in counseling does not necessarily mean a single-session. Clients are routinely invited to return for a subsequent walk-in session or to make an appointment for further services. Some return and some do not. However, with a walk-in mindset, therapists are always thinking that the current session is potentially the final one. We organize our sessions with that thought in mind and strive to be maximally effective in every session. We expect our students to be aware that many clients will not return. They learn that many of our clients come to counseling expecting to have only one session and that some clients are surprised and disappointed when asked to make further appointments. Often, it is the therapists, rather than the clients, who expect therapy to continue after an initial session.

The following assumptions, borrowed from O'Hanlon & Weiner-Davis (1989), serve to reinforce a single-session mindset:

1. Rapid change is not only possible, but common in human experience.
2. Therapists' expectations are communicated overtly and covertly about how rapid and how much change can be expected.
3. There is no direct correlation between the duration of the complaint and the duration of the treatment.

4. There is no direct correlation between the severity of the complaint and the duration of the treatment.
5. We need to know less about the history of the complaint and the person than we think.
6. Clients are far less interested in psychotherapy than are therapists.
7. The greatest opportunity for change comes in the earliest stages of therapy.

We also want our students to understand that longer is not necessarily better. Here are some of the reasons:

- One session is often the client's preferred number of sessions. When therapists conduct their sessions with that timeframe in mind, many clients will be appreciative, and the therapeutic alliance will be strengthened.
- By communicating to clients that one session can make a significant difference, we are indirectly letting clients know that we have confidence in them. This is empowering.
- When therapy lasts a long time, clients and their significant others may come to assume that the problems are severe.
- In our time-sensitive world, the briefer the therapy the less disruptive to everyday life. Clients miss less work, school, or leisure activities.
- One session of therapy is less financially burdensome for clients.
- For nonprofit service providers, completing therapy in one session is highly cost-efficient, enables more clients to be served with the same resources, and reduces wait lists.

Description of The Context

In each of the contexts in which we provided walk-in counseling, we employed a team approach. Typically, a team consists of three to six therapists along with a supervisor (sometimes called shift coordinator). The therapists may be mental health professionals employed by an agency, graduate students receiving training, or professionals who volunteer their time as a form of contribution to their community or as a further learning experience. In some instances, a co-therapy model is used in which two therapists jointly conduct the interview. In other instances it is a solo therapist. In either case, the supervisor and other team members watch the therapy session from behind a one-way mirror or via closed circuit television. The observing team members occasionally make suggestions by telephone during the session. The team meets toward the end of the session to compare observations and plan interventions.

When clients first walk in, they are greeted in a respectful manner and wait in a comfortable waiting area. We want our clients to be as relaxed as possible before the session begins. The team receives the forms that clients completed in the waiting room and prepares one or two of the team members to conduct the session. These forms include some brief demographic data, a description of the problem using solution-focused prompts, permission or denial to participate with a team behind the mirror, and a self-determined presession measure of distress marked on a 10-point scale. Examples of possible questions for a walk-in intake form are found in Table 1. Sometimes, the reception or intake staff will also share observations about the clients. During this presession the team very tentatively, based on the forms that have been completed, begins to speculate about what the clients might want from the session

Table 1
Examples of Questions for a Walk-in Intake Form

1. What is the single most important concern that you would like to discuss today?

2. What would be important for us to know about the background of this concern?

3. If 10 is the best and 1 is the worst, how are things in your life today?
   Worst 1 2 3 4 5 6 7 8 9 10 Best

4. Have you had previous counseling? Yes / No
   What was most / least useful about it?

5. What would someone else come to admire and respect most about you if they had months or years to get to know you? It's OK to guess.

6. What would someone else come to admire and respect most about your child / children if they had months or years to get to know them? It's OK to guess.

7. For many people, a single session with a counselor is sufficient to take a first step. What would be the smallest change that would tell you that you are headed in the right direction?

In some settings, the presession measure is the Session Rating Scale (SRS) and the post-session rating scale is the Outcome Rating Scale (ORS) developed by Duncan, Miller, Sparks, Claud, Reynolds, Brown, & Johnson (2003).

and how to give it to them. These speculations give the therapist a beginning focus for the session.

Each session is 50 minutes in length and is organized using the five-part Milan model (Boscolo et. al., 1987), i.e. presession, session, intersession, intervention delivery (which we commonly refer to as "feedback from the team") and postsession. The conversation with the client (the session) is about 30 minutes in length and is observed by the therapy team. The therapist takes a break to consult with the team and to develop team feedback (the intersession). The therapist returns to the client, delivers the team's feedback to the client, and responds to any responses that the client may have. (Note: The delivery of the intervention might also take the form of a reflecting team (Andersen, 1987) whereby the team behind the mirror goes in front while the client and therapist go behind the mirror and hear the team hypothesize about the client's situation and offer commendations and suggestions.) At the end of the session, the team debriefs (postsession).

Before clients leave the center, the therapist asks them to complete a feedback form that includes a postsession measure of distress as well as questions that invite the client to address how and if the session met their needs. We take this feedback seriously. Any negative feedback is addressed with the client, usually before they leave the session.

A Walk-in Therapy Practice Framework

We begin this discussion with a set of underlying tenets that set the stage for our therapeutic principles. This is followed by the how to's of our practice framework. Appendix A provides a summary format for walk-in sessions.

UNDERLYING TENETS

It's just one hour: The fact that the entire therapy takes place in one hour, with no prior information available to the therapist and no follow-up to the session, plays a major role in how this service is clinically conceptualized. The importance of the therapeutic alliance cannot be underestimated; in a walk-in session the therapist has little time to spare in building a sufficient alliance. Historical fishing expeditions are ruled out; there is not enough time. Therapists who typically begin their sessions with a multi-generational genogram may, in the interest of time, rethink their usual approach in favor of one that more quickly focuses on presenting concerns.

Clients who present multiple issues can be a particular challenge. For these clients, therapists need to hone skills in negotiating a focus that is achievable in one hour by asking, for example, "What is most important today?" or by selecting a common theme that encompasses each of the presenting concerns. The questions a therapist chooses to ask must be carefully considered through a lens that takes time into account. One "innocent" question could lead to twenty minutes of conversation that is not helpful in assisting clients to focus on what they want from today's session.

The one-hour time frame also means that therapists must hone their skills at redirecting clients who have long stories to tell. Clients need to be heard, but it may be necessary to gently remind them about the 50-minute timeframe so they can make choices about which aspects of their story are important for the therapist to know. One colleague positions a large clock on the wall directly behind him. He then mentions the time at which he will take his break to consult with his team and asks the client to let him know when they reach that time. In that way, the client and therapist share responsibility for how the time unfolds.

We narrow the database: Fisch (1994) argues that the narrower the database of the therapeutic conversation, the shorter the therapy. Like Fisch, therapists who conduct walk-in sessions guide the session in such a way as to shorten conversation time. They do this by focusing on the problem as it occurs in the present. It follows that walk-in therapists guide the discussion towards current and future (as opposed to past) data with a particular interest in descriptive (as opposed to explanatory) data. For example, the therapist is interested in who, what, when, how and with whom a youth's disrespectful behavior occurs. The therapist does not focus on questions about the youth's past, theories of underlying cause, or the function of the problem. We borrow from Solution Focused and Narrative therapists (Berg & Miller, 1992; Freedman & Coombs, 1996; Lipchik, 2002; White, 1986; White & Epston 1990) in assuming that "the problem is the problem" as the client presents it. Assuming underlying causes, pathology within the individual, or unconscious motivations can prolong therapy. Instead, the focus is on problems as aspects of human interaction. Assuming that change requires insight can prolong therapy; viewing change as involving the client doing some kind of task will shorten it. Establishing specific goals described in behavioral terms enables therapists and clients to efficiently focus and structure the session.

It's a whole therapy: We begin each session assuming that this session is the whole therapy. This idea is well captured by the following statement from Ray & Keeney (1993), though not written specifically about single-session or walk-in therapy:

> All sessions aim at being a whole therapy. This helps create a focus on achieving a beginning, middle and end. Should the clients return for a subsequent session, that session is treated as a new case. Of course, the

> new case will have to consider the session that took place with the other therapist the time before. That other therapist, who might be you at another time, will have to be considered now as part of the therapy. (p.12)

The idea that each session is a whole therapy may seem like a radical idea to some therapists. However, it can also serve as a reminder that many, if not most, clients are fans of brief therapy. One session, if they believe that it helped, is the best therapy of all.

Common factors: Meta-analyses of four decades of psychotherapy outcome research have supported the conclusion that while psychotherapy is effective for most clients, that effectiveness is not due to the uniqueness of the various models of therapy but rather to factors that are shared by all psychotherapy models (Hubble, Duncan and Miller, 1999; Duncan, Miller & Sparks, 2004; Wampold, 2001). Brown, Dreis and Nace (1999) say this about successful outcomes: "Seventy percent of the total outcome variance is accounted for when a strong therapeutic relationship is combined with a successful incorporation of client factors in the treatment process" (p.309). According to these analyses of the research literature, a strong therapeutic alliance is based on good listening, expressions of empathy and support, and client perception that there is a good fit between the therapists methods of conducting therapy (the model) and the client's own ideas about what will work for him or her. When that strong alliance utilizes already existing client strengths, resources and beliefs, successful outcomes are likely. Thus, in our walk-in sessions, we strive to assist clients to make use of their client's system resources, attend to client motivation, focus on client wants, and link hope with expectations for improvement from the therapeutic process. Simultaneously, we seek continuous feedback from the client about whether the procedures (the model) used by the therapist are a good fit.

Therapeutic influences are tempered with pragmatism: Those of us who have been involved in the development of this framework subscribe to a variety of therapeutic influences that share certain meta-theoretical, philosophic threads. These include systemic, postmodern, social constructionist and Ericksonian ideas. The work of the Mental Research Institute (MRI) (Fisch, Weakland, Segal, & Fisch, 1982; Watzlawick, Weakland, & Fisch, 1974) and the solution focused therapists (De Shazer, 1985; O'Hanlon & Weiner-Davis, 1989; Walter & Peller, 1992) contributed to our thinking. Those two closely related approaches have long been associated with brief therapy. Other models that have contributed to our ideas include Narrative (White & Epston, 1990; Freedman & Combs, 1996) and Strategic (Haley, 1973; Madanes, 1982). However, consistent with postmodern thought, no model is considered more correct than another. Our primary interest is in what is useful for this client at this point in time. Therefore, models of therapy that do not usually fit within the above philosophical threads, such as Cognitive Behaviour Therapy, may be a good fit for some clients at some points in time (Young, 2008 p. 34; Schoener, 5). Any approach can work that can be made to fit within the constraints of a "whole therapy" in one hour, especially if the approach is acceptable to the client. Ours is essentially a pragmatic perspective (Amundson, 1996).

The session is a consultation: We prefer to think of walk-in therapy as a consultation process in which the therapist offers ideas (many of which may have come from the client), and the client decides whether to accept them, reject them, or put them on hold. Clients leave the session and may or may not make use of the therapeutic conversation. It's up to them. Often, the therapist has no long-term feedback from the clients about the outcomes. The consultation stance helps therapists to resist the temptation to take responsibility for client change. We believe that the client is his own greatest resource and is in the best position to evaluate the ideas generated during the session. Our job is to create a context that enables the client to discover those resources and teach us how to be their guide.

THE MODEL IN ACTION

The goal of a walk-in therapy session differs with each client. However, in a generic sense, our goal in walk-in therapy is for the client to leave the session with a sense of emotional relief, increased hope, and some sort of positive outcome as defined by the client. For one client, a positive outcome may be as straightforward as knowing that someone has heard and validated their story. For another client it could be a new way of thinking about a problem—the beginning of a new story. A new way of thinking about a problem, in another instance, may involve deciding that this situation is not a problem after all. Another client may leave the session with a specific task, a new way of approaching a troubling issue. Or a client may leave with ideas about where to get further help. We achieve these outcomes by focusing on the following ideas.

What does the client want? We want to learn, as early as possible, what the client wants from the session. We might ask: "What are you hoping for from today's meeting? or "What needs to happen during our time together that will make you feel that it was worth your while to come here today?" (Note the use of the word "today" in these questions. This plants a seed for the client that our plan is to make today's session work for them.) Answering this question is an opportunity for the client to guide the therapist. The therapist can then focus on this goal and avoid "snipe hunts" that do not address the client's immediate concern. A client recently began a session by saying, "I've seen two psychiatrists and three psychologists and none of them let me talk." This client was saying to the therapist, "just listen", so that is exactly what the therapist did for the entire session. At the end of the session, the therapist asked if the session was helpful. The client said she was greatly relieved. The first step is learning what the client wants. The remainder of the session is about giving that to the client.

It is important to note that what the client wants may be unrelated to the presenting concern. For example, one depressed client might want a referral for medication while another might want to develop new goals for herself.

Developing a contextual understanding: We find a useful question that helps to narrow the database is "why now?" Why has this parent, who has been struggling for three years to get her son to get to school on time, decided to come for a session on this particular evening? The answer to this question can help the therapist to put context to the problem and to place the problem in present interactions. The answer might tell us, for example, that the school is threatening a suspension. Or, perhaps mother and son had a physical altercation that morning as the mother tried to get her son out of bed. Or, perhaps the divorced father is threatening a custody battle by saying that the son's lateness is a sign of the mother's inadequate parenting. Each answer to the "why now" question provides different ideas to the therapist about the next questions to be asked. Other contextual questions could be:

- How is this a problem for you now?
- Why did you choose to come today?
- Who else is aware of your situation?
- If your spouse/partner were here, what would he say about your situation?
- Who in your life would be most affected if the problem disappeared?

Client Resources: We adhere strongly to the notion that only clients can solve their problems, and all clients have resources that can be directed toward problem solving. The job of the therapist is to direct the conversation in such a way that resources that could be used for problem solving are mutually discovered. Questions could include:

- What have you done to prevent the problem from completely taking over your life?
- How have others in your life been helpful to you?
- What has worked even a little bit in the past?
- What has given you the strength to endure?
- What would family members, friends, or co-workers say are your greatest assets?

Client resources might include the personal resources of the individual client as well as the resources of the client's social network (family, friends, work colleagues, teachers, etc). It is not unusual, for example, for a session to focus on how to ask a friend for assistance or how to invite a family member to accompany the client to a future walk-in session.

Attempted solutions: Sometimes, consistent with the work of the MRI (Watzlawick, Weakland and Fisch, 1988), we find it useful to consider the notion that "the problem is the attempted solution." We want to learn what the client has tried in the past that has not worked and, equally important, what attempted solutions have worked, even if just a little bit, for a short period of time. At minimum, we do not want to disempower ourselves or the client by suggesting something that has not worked before. At best, by making use of a previously attempted positive solution, we might introduce a small change that successfully addresses the presenting concern.

In a recent walk-in session at the Austin Guidance Center, Austin, Texas, an 11-year old girl and her mother presented with the problem of the girl's refusal to attend school due to anxiety. In an attempt to deal with the issue, the mother had been driving her to school in the morning, but the girl refused to enter the school even when her teacher offered to walk her from the car to the classroom. After the therapist learned that the girl was doing well academically and had good relationships with her classmates and teachers, the following was suggested. The therapist told the mother and daughter that while it is unfortunate that fear was getting the better of the daughter, it was most important for the daughter to see that her mother could stand up to the daughter's fear. Therefore, the mother was asked to take her previous attempted solution (driving her daughter to school) one step further by accompanying her daughter to the classroom, even holding her hand if necessary, "to give your daughter comfort and support." The mother was to stay in the classroom for as long as her daughter indicated that her mother was needed. This intervention was designed to a) build on the mother's previous attempted solution of driving her daughter to school, b) take advantage of the mother's schedule which allowed her the time to do this, and c) motivate this 11-year old to get to school on her own in order to avoid the embarrassment of having her mother sit with her in class.

An example of an attempted solution is when a client tells us about something that has helped during a past difficulty; then that might be highlighted and the client encouraged to apply that solution to the present concern. For example, a client could be encouraged to use a simple self-care strategy that has worked before, such as taking a warm bath, going for a walk, or phoning a friend.

One aspect of the attempted solutions question that bears particular mention is learning about previous professional assistance. When a client reports that previous therapy has been helpful, we want to know what in particular was helpful, because we may want to build on the work of the previous therapist. There is an anecdote about a therapist who asked for advice from one of the founders of the Strategic Therapy model, Jay Haley, when a family the therapist had seen five years before returned with the same problem. After learning what the therapist had done five years earlier, Haley is reported to have said: "Do it again; it worked for five years!" Thus, we may want to take advantage of what has worked before rather than attempt something new and untested.

Occasionally, a client who comes to a walk-in service is actively involved in treatment with another mental health professional. Unless the client is highly dissatisfied with that professional, we will ask the client to describe the work she is doing in that other treatment so that we can use the present session to support that work.

Making use of client motivation: We do not adhere to the concept of resistance in our walk-in therapy work. We agree with de Shazer (1986) that it is best to think in terms of client-therapist cooperation and that it is the therapist's responsibility to build a cooperative relationship. We believe that all clients are motivated. Therefore, we attend closely to what motivates clients to attend their walk-in session. Some clients attend because they want help in solving problems. Some come in order to complain about someone else. Some feel coerced by others (parent, probation officer).

Some models of therapy (e.g., SFT, MRI) have given particular attention to the question of how to turn lack of cooperation into cooperation. We utilize those ideas as well as the work of Prochaska and DiClemente (1982) on client readiness for change. Our neophyte practitioners of walk-in therapy tell us that by focusing on client readiness and the therapist-client relationship, they learn to avoid producing resistance by not doing more than the client wants them to do.

Think small: Many clients who attend walk-in sessions have experienced a recent crisis. It helps in those situations to compress time. This can be done by "anchoring the pain in the immediate past, presupposing that today is different, that it is better…" (Lipchick, 2002). The session then becomes a search for small changes, such as "How did you get out of bed today and come to this session?" In this approach, we believe change is constant and that small change leads to big change. An end of session task might be to ask that client to do one small self-care act in the next 24 hours. Therapists who think small take pressure off of themselves and do not make the error of promoting more change than the client wants.

Solution Focused Therapy (SFT): Solution Focused Therapy (deShazer,

1986; Berg & Dolan, 2001) introduced a number of clinical interviewing techniques that we find useful in walk-in sessions. These ideas are designed to move clients away from focusing primarily on the problem and toward focusing on solutions. Some of these ideas include: attending to exceptions to the problem (already existing periods when the problem is not occurring); future oriented questions (what the client might be doing once the problem is not dominating his/her life); developing focused goals; scaling questions ("If the problem intensity is currently rated as a 6 on a 10 point scale, what needs to happen to reduce the problem to a 5?"); and coping questions ("In spite of the problem, how is it that you are doing as well as your are?"). We invite the reader to review the Solution SFT references named above for further explication of these techniques.

Client theory of change: According to Duncan & Miller (2000):

> Because all approaches are equivalent with respect to outcome, and technique pales in comparison to client and relationship factors, an evolving story casts the client as not only the star of the therapeutic stage, but also the director of the change process. We now consider our clients' worldviews, their maps of the territory, as the determining "theory", directing both the destination desired and the routes of restoration (p.78).

In walk-in therapy, we invite clients to guide us in how to be most helpful to them. We do this by asking them what they want from the therapy process, their beliefs about the problem ("theory of the problem"), and their ideas about what would help ("theory of change"). Examples of questions might be:

- What will work for you *today*?
- Are there any questions that you wish to ask that I did not get to?
- For many people, a single-session with a therapist is sufficient to take action; what would be the smallest step that would tell you that you are headed in the right direction?

A mother and her 15-year-old son recently came for a walk-in session. The mother, convinced that her son had been unhappy since the parents' separation, explained that she had taken her son to numerous therapists, and he had not liked any of them. The son, who looked sullen and had not spoken until that point, said, "I liked one." He then spoke of how he had been helped by a therapist who told stories about the therapist's own family. The boy was invited to ask the therapist any questions he wanted, even if they were personal. The mother watched as the boy had an animated, though abstract, discussion with the therapist about family life. Mother and son left in much better spirits with the mother saying they would return, "If we need to."

Commendations: After taking an inter-session break, the therapist returns to share solution oriented ideas from the therapy team. Prior to offering solutions the therapist offers commendations from the team (McElheran & Harper-Jaques, 1994; Houger Limacher, 2003). These are positive statements of what the team has noticed about the client/family. These commendations serve several purposes:

- They highlight strengths and resources that the client may not have noticed and thereby may point the way toward solutions.
- They positively surprise those clients who expect to be criticized for their missteps and mistakes.
- They relax clients, making them more receptive to the team's recommendations.

Case Example: The Girl Who Cried

This session took place at the Community Counseling Service (CCS) of Our Lady of the Lake University (Chapter 7). It is located in a low Socioeconomic Status (SES), largely Latino area of San Antonio, Texas. Clients are seen either by appointment or by walking in. The CCS provides training to masters and doctoral counseling psychology students. It utilizes a team format in which six graduate students work with a faculty supervisor. Ordinarily, two graduate students working as co-therapists interview the client(s) while the team and supervisor observe through closed circuit television. Part way through the session the therapists take a break and consult with the team. The therapists then return to the clients and provide feedback from the team.

In the transcript below, we (Arnie Slive and Monte Bobele) agreed to conduct the session as a demonstration for the students. Carmen and her daughter Julia, age 11, had scheduled this appointment a few days earlier. They are Mexican-Americans who lived within a couple of miles of the CCS. Although this was not a walk-in session, it serves to exemplify many of the principles of walk in therapy. For the purposes of this discussion about our walk-in model, the transcript is not chronological but is divided into key themes.

The transcript that follows, which has been edited to fit within the space confines of this chapter, uses pseudonyms for the clients.

Problem Description

Monte: We have a piece of paper here that tells us just a little bit about why you called for an appointment, but we don't have a whole lot of information.

Carmen: Uh-huh. Well, the reason is I've been having a little bit of problems with her as far as she gets very irritable. It's been going on for a while, but it's just been getting a little bit worse as far as she just finds like reasons to cry. Like she has a little two-year-old brother. And she'll just cry for hours. And she'll—I try to reason with her. She just blocks everything out that you say.

Monte: Really? Wow.

Carmen: She won't listen. She just, cries, and she just can't stop. And it just goes on about at least once a week, at least. You know, it just didn't seem normal, so—it just—it's been going on for so often. It's just very easy to make her cry. And she just—I—you can't stop her. She has to stop on her own.

Arnie: So one thing that would probably help us is if you could recall an instance of crying. Take us through that. You know, sort of describe what happened.

Carmen: Okay. Well, she has a two-year-old little brother. And, of course, they have little disagreements and stuff. So I'll tell her just, "Behave," or "Don't be fighting with him." And, she'll get upset, and she'll just cry. And then she'll just run straight to her room, slam her door, and just cry. It'll be around noontime, and she won't stop crying till about three o'clock or so…And, she'll just be crying and crying. I can go in there. I'll let her for a little bit. And, I'll go over there and say, "What's wrong?" And it's just like if I'm not there. So it's just—she'll --

Monte: So it's like she can't hear you.

Carmen: Like—yeah. She completely—but, she just cries and cries. And I try to reason with her, and everything. And I—I do things with her and—I don't neglect her. We do things on the weekends. We—you know, whatever. So I try to give them both that equal attention so she wouldn't, get upset. But, she just—I just took her out and stuff, and it happened that day. She just—later on, she got into a little argument with her brother, her little brother. And she just ran to her room and just cried. And it was just something very little, and she just cried for hours. And I just asked her if anything's bothering her besides that, because it seemed a little more than just that. And she said "no." Or—well, later on she said "no." But she just kept crying and crying and crying.

Monte: How did that come to an end, after three hours of crying?

Here is a first attempt to move toward a focus on potential solutions.

Carmen: Her grandma went in there for a little bit, later on after she just—she gets tired, and she just—she find a point where she's—you can tell she's kind of simmering down. And then you have to go and—but when she first starts out, there's just no way you can talk to her.

Arnie: And sometimes you or her grandma, or somebody, is with her, and sometimes she's just alone in her room?

Carmen: First—first, we'll go check on her and see if there's any way we can get through to her. But then if we can't, we just leave her alone and just let her cry it out. Because sometimes if you try, it just makes it worse. She just cries more.

Arnie: Like for her whole—I can understand how, like you say, at the end that she's just tired, because it takes a lot of stamina—to cry for that long.

Carmen: And it just—can't get through to her. It's just—you just want to know why.

Later in the session…

Carmen: But then there's just instances where she'll just find a reason to cry. Like she knows I'm going to tell her no about something, and then she'll just—run out crying, because she knows—

Monte: Oh. So she knows even before you tell her no that you're going to say "no."

Carmen: You know, and then she just does it so—because she knows it's going to upset me. And then she'll just run in her room crying—and then I'll try to go and console her and tell her, "You know, we talked about it. I already told you, wait till next week," or whichever, you know. And then she just—she don't respond.

Monte: You haven't given up yet. But, you're really trying hard to be a good mom.

Carmen: I try, but sometimes I think the best thing is just to leave her alone and just let her cry it out. And she just falls asleep. And then later—that's the only way that she'll—because if you try sometimes to talk to her, she just gets worse or [unintelligible] just leave her alone, and then she'll just cry it out 'til she falls asleep. And then when she gets up, she'll just be like—you could talk to her then.

Arnie: Well, when—okay. So when she gets up, after she's had a sleep. And do you talk with her right after she gets up, or do you wait a while to talk to her?

Carmen: Later on, after she's cried it out, then she—she'll be like, "Okay," or now she understands. But we could have avoided the whole crying situation if she would have just listened. But she just—she will just cry.

Arnie: But it is—it does sound, to me, like—I'm not sure what you think about this, but it does sound to me—it's like it's a good thing that she does eventually get to that place where you and she can have a conversation about it, and where she can be—you can tell her—explain your reasoning to her—and that she can accept that, that she does eventually get to that place.

Carmen: Eventually, yeah.

Notice that our questions are primarily focused on understanding the problem in the present. There is little discussion of the past.

Why now?

In our experience, there is usually a precipitating event that leads a client to initiate counseling. Sometimes this event is a sign that the problem is beyond the client's previously used coping strategies. Sometime clients arrive at our door because someone else has recently referred them. Understanding the circumstances of the current session is important.

Monte: Has it gotten worse? Is that why --

Carmen: It just started being more frequent.

Monte: More frequent?

Carmen: Yeah. I mean, she's had some pretty bad episodes. We were at my boyfriend's apartment one time, and people live downstairs, and they actually thought that we were abusing her, because she was crying so much and making so much noise—that they went upstairs and said, "What's going on here?"

What do the clients want from the session?

As stated earlier, giving the clients what they want is an important consideration for single-session therapy. We want to establish the clients' goals for the visit as early as possible.

Monte: So when you called to make the appointment to come here, what were you hoping that we could help you and Julia with?

Carmen: Just figure out a reason why? Is this normal? Or is this—what—why does it—because I know there's other 11-year-olds, and they don't do that, so—

Later in the session…

Carmen: I just don't think it's normal for someone to cry for three hours at a time. It's just—and I just want to know if there's any other—why is that? Or is there any way I can help that or—?

Still later in the session...

Arnie: So you'd like for this to happen less often and not for as long. But it—and I just want to check this with you, if I'm right about what I'm hearing, that the main thing is not that she cries, but that she cries for so long?

Carmen: Yeah. I just—well, I'd prefer she didn't cry for so long or even cry for any little thing that just—I want to know what the real cause of it is. You know, maybe there's—I don't know.

Monte: So there's some times if Julia was crying and you knew what it was all about, you wouldn't be quite so concerned, like if she fell down?

Carmen: Yeah. That's the thing.

Monte: So those times when—if her brother accidentally hits her or something like that, and she starts crying, you're not worried about—that, because you just said it's just a normal girl....

Carmen: And it doesn't go on for a long time.

And still later...

Arnie: So you're here because you want to know if there's something seriously wrong.

Carmen: Well, I just—yeah, and, I mean—if it's not, then that's fine, and it's not just—it's normal, and I just [unintelligible] there's other help or she needs something, I can at least get her treated to find a solution to stop that, because I don't want her to be like that. She's getting bigger, and she's getting older and, you know.

Arnie: And when you think about getting treated, do you have some ideas about that?

Carmen: No. I don't even know where to start on that. I just—that's why—I mean, if it's normal and stuff, then I'll just—okay, you know. But I just don't think it is, but—

Arnie: And if it were normal, what do you think you would do then? If you came to really believe that it was normal, what would you do? How would you handle it?

Carmen: [unintelligible] just, you know—she's going to continue. It's her habit. It's her behavior. There's just nothing I can do about it.

Arnie: It's just something about who she is—

Frequently, the answer to the question of what the client wants evolves during the session. In this session it began with a desire to understand why. It evolved to include the question of whether this is a serious problem and wanting to learn what could be done to help.

ENGAGING JULIA

Arnie: Julia, if I could just ask you. What did you think about coming today? Whose idea was it to come here?

Julia: [unintelligible]
Carmen: She's really shy.
Arnie: Mm-hmm. Well, was it more your idea? Was it more your mom's idea?
Julia: My mom's idea.
Monte: What did she tell you about coming here today?
Julia: She just told me what to do.
Monte: I wonder if Julia is shy with everybody, or if she's just shy with strangers like us and warms up to people after a while.
Carmen: Yeah. She's shy at first. This is new to her, so she's a little nervous.

(A period of awkward silence)

Arnie: *(to Monte)* So there's a good chance that she has friends that she's not shy with at all.
Monte: That she talks with on the phone or plays with.
Carmen: No. She don't talk on the phone. And she plays with little kids.

The challenge of engaging Julia was present throughout the session. The above dialogue was her entire verbalization. Julia rarely made eye contact and several times covered her head with her hooded sweatshirt. Although we could have seen her alone for part of the session, we elected not to because we were concerned that would be even more intimidating to her.

Diagnostic questions

In this portion of the interview, we want to explore what explanations Carmen may already have heard or considered about Julia's condition.
Carmen: I know she is on medication for her heart, so I don't know. It might—maybe it's, you know, kind of making her mood changes and stuff.
Monte: Really? How long has she been on the heart medicine?
Carmen: For about four years.
Monte: Okay. And so the crying was—did she have these crying episodes before her brother was born?
Carmen: Yes. Yes.
Monte: And, before the medicine?
Carmen: Not as much, not really.
Arnie: Who is it that prescribes the medicine?
Carmen: Her cardiologist.
Arnie: And is it something that you've talked with the cardiologist about?
Carmen: I've spoken to him. He said it shouldn't affect her moods, so—

Monte: What's she like when she's not here with strangers? When she's at home with her family or her friends?

Carmen: Oh, she's fine. You know, she—she'll look at TV. She'll play with her brother, fight with her brother, back and forth. And she likes to go to her room a lot and just play by herself. She has, her dollhouse and stuff, so she'll just—she'll be alone for a while.

Arnie: And how's school going?

Carmen: School's going fine. She takes special classes in school, so—and right now she's passing them, so far. But she gets help in everything.

Later in the session...

Monte: Well, I was thinking there's one other thing that might be helpful in understanding this. Sometimes people cry because they're sad.... And, Carmen, is it your sense that, for the most part, she's a happy child, and once in a while she starts crying? Or, is she sad and cries on top of that?

Carmen: I don't know if she's sad. I mean, I try to do everything. I mean, I do what I can for her. Whatever she wants, I buy it for her and—and I ask her if she has any problems at school. She says "no." I always ask her how's school—if anything's wrong, talk to me or—she's got some moments where she's just real quiet, and she doesn't talk to anybody. And I ask her, "Are you okay?" She says, "Yes."

Monte: So, she's not sad most of the time.

Carmen: Most of the time, no.

Monte: Yeah. Okay. So just—it sounds like when she cries, it's more—almost a more angry or frustrated cry than a—

Carmen: Yeah.

One of the principles that we follow is: continue to narrow the database on information that we have to work with. Within our single-session mindset, this means that we make constant choices about the questions to ask, including diagnostic questions. We chose to briefly explore the cardiac medication issue and the question of depression. We chose not to explore her cardiac condition. We also took note of, but did not explore the possibility that, Julia has significant learning/developmental issues. For example, we learned that she plays with younger children and she attends special classes, but we did not delve into that area. These issues may have been a factor in Julia's silence throughout the session. These therapeutic choices are based on what the clients want from the session and what we believe will be the most useful information to help us to address those wants.

Attempted solutions

Arnie: There was something you said a couple minutes ago I wanted to ask you about. You said sometimes you think maybe the best thing to do is just to leave her? Let her cry, just leave her?

Carmen: Yeah, because there's no way I can get to her.

Arnie: Right! Exactly. So have there been times when you've said "no" about something, she becomes upset, starts to cry, goes to her room, and you've just left her for the whole time, for as long as she needs to do that, without going to her, without talking to her? Or, without her grandmother talking to her? Have there been—have you ever done that?

Carmen: Have I ever done—? I think I've done it once. And, she started, kicking her doors, and throwing stuff. And so I had to go over there and see what's [unintelligible]—

Arnie: Like, kind of like a tantrum, you mean?

Carmen: Yeah, kind of like getting—trying to get my attention or—because I was like, "Okay. Well, just—I'll just leave her alone." And she'll be crying and crying, crying. And I'm like, "I'm just going to let her," you know, thinking it's going to stop, because she's going to realize, you know—but then she just throws stuff or kicks something, and that's where I have to go over there and say—

Monte: What would happen if you didn't?

Carmen: If I didn't go?

Monte: If you didn't go over there when she was kicking and throwing things?

Carmen: She probably would break something in her room or something.

Monte: What might be the first thing she'd break?

Carmen: I don't know, probably her—she has dollhouses or something or—I don't know. She'll kick the walls or something, just to make noise. It doesn't matter, just—she'll do anything just to make noise that is banging something or—

Monte: Okay. Are you—when you want to stop her from doing that, are you worried she's going to hurt herself from kicking the walls? Are you worried?

Carmen: Well, yeah. I'm worried. But—yeah, I'm worried. But most of the time, I'll try to either wait, go and see what's wrong, and—try, even though most of the time it's not successful. But I'll try. I try anyways.

Later in the session we explore the social context and other things she has tried.

Monte: Is it your mother that lives with you?

Carmen: Yeah. It's my mom.

Monte: Does she have any advice about this?

Carmen: She's tried the talking to her. Tried leaving her alone. And, my mom likes to give in to her more than I would. But, I'm the one that's like, "No, I can't do that. I already did this," or whichever. My mom's more like, "Oh, well, she's going to get mad. She's going to start crying." I'm—

Monte: Yeah. So grandmothers are kind of like that, huh?

At this point we interrupted the session to consult with the team. The team thought that the first part of the session had already begun to address one of Carmen's reasons for coming to therapy: the question of why does this happen. We had begun to co-construct new meanings to Julia's behavior by referring to it as tantrums and as expressions of anger or frustration. Tantrums and anger are the kinds of problems parents can become experts in helping their children eliminate. We hoped to reduce Carmen's worry that Julia had serious emotional problems, but instead, had normal childhood problems. Therefore, the team focused primarily on addressing the question of whether this is a serious problem and on how to help Carmen and Julia with new ideas for addressing the crying spells.

After the break.

Commendations

The first thing we want to do after a team break is to provide some feedback, or an assessment, to the clients. We focus on strengths and assets identified in the first part of the session. We begin by commending Carmen and Julia.

Arnie: Well, first of all, everyone—we all wanted to share with you, Carmen, that we think you're a really great mom.

Carmen: Oh, thank you.

Arnie: It's obvious that the two of you have a close relationship. That Julia will talk with you about—She feels that you're somebody that she can talk to about things.

Carmen: Mm-hmm.

Arnie: She's doing well in her life. You're highly committed. And just the fact of your coming here—it's just like this is what a good parent would do. I mean, something that feels unusual to you has been happening, and you just want to check that out.

Carmen: Yeah.

Monte: It wouldn't be unusual for some parents to say, "I'm just going to ignore it and not pay attention to it." But you're really concerned about her, and that shows. And, even though she doesn't talk much, we can tell from the way she looks at you that she really feels close to you and trusts you.

Carmen: Yeah.

Monte: And she can hide her eyes so that we won't be able to see that, but we saw it before.

Arnie: But, I've noticed a twinkle in her eye, too.

The intervention/homework

There have been ongoing conversations in the literature about interventions. This chapter is not the place to review or comment on this debate. We think every session needs to end with some sort of reflection, task, homework, or suggestion. We also recognize the irony of assigning tasks to clients when there is little or no expectation that they will return. Frequently, these assignments are characterized as potentially useful if or when the client may return. In this case, we formulated a task based on the likelihood that Carmen and Julia would not be planning to return in the near future.

Arnie: So, based on our conversation, we're not in a position to say, "Well, it's this, it's that." We're leaning in the direction of saying that this is not a highly unusual problem. This is what our thinking is, without saying—we can't say this is a certainty. Our thinking is that this—that there's some things that you could try out—that could provide us with a little bit more information that could help us to be clearer and more certain about that—that this is not a—a big, problem that needs—that somebody's going to need, years of treatment or something like that.

Carmen: Yeah.

Arnie: But, we feel it would be good just to get a little bit more information.

Carmen: Uh-huh.

Monte: I'm wondering if you—do you think—would you be willing to try a couple of things, small things, to help us understand the situation better?

Carmen: Okay. What is—

Mom's hesitancy to say yes is seen as a positive sign—the response of someone who is seriously thinking about what is being presented.

Arnie: Well, we're thinking about—so this is something that—I mean, there's a couple of things. One is that what Julia has been doing with these episodes would be difficult for any parent.

Carmen: Yeah.

Arnie: I mean, you love your daughter, and you're—it worries you. And, it's hard on her, too.

Carmen: Yeah.

Arnie: And, so some ideas that could help you to manage it when it does happen—and also to help her to begin to learn how—a little bit more about how to manage herself when she's feeling frustrated.

Carmen: Yeah.

Arnie: You know? So this is what we're thinking—is if you think about this as an experiment.

Carmen: Mm-hmm.

Arnie: If over the next while, the next couple of times that this happens—if, when one of these occasions happens where something's happening, she wants something, you say "no" and the crying begins—and this—I recognize this could be hard—that you just let it happen. Let her do what she's going to do, like go to her room, cry, be upset, but just not get involved. Okay? I know you'll hear it happening. I'm not saying you're not going to be feeling concerned about it. But that you just will let it happen, not—not get involved—until it finishes.

With almost every phrase, mom says, "Mm-hmm."

Monte: *(to Arnie)* It might even be helpful if she'd make note about how long this happens from start to finish. That would be very important—to get an accurate timing on this.

Arnie: And any other observations that you have during—

Carmen: Oh, okay.

Arnie: So when—how long it happens. It might be good to put down the date that it happens—

Carmen: Yeah.

Arnie: The time of day, how long it happens, and then any other—any—just anything else that you think is important to note.

Carmen: Okay.

Monte: Maybe even what they were talking about before it happened.

Carmen: The whole—okay.

Monte: Can you do that?

Carmen: Yeah.

Arnie: And then afterwards—okay—when you get together, I—I think it would be nice—you could get together over some milk and cookies and talk about what happened. Okay? Just the two of you.

Carmen: Yeah.

Arnie: So you could have a chat, the two of you. And you could make some notes about that too, about that conversation and what she told you about what was going on for her.

Carmen: Yeah. I can do that.

Arnie: And if you get concerned—you were saying before, "Well, she'd kick things or hurt things." What we would say is that the only reason that you would get involved is if you thought she was doing harm to herself.

Carmen: Oh, okay.

Arnie: But other than that—even if something does break—You know, I mean, toys or whatever that break—well, they're not people—it's too bad, but—and we'd also recommend that you speak with her grandmother about it, just so she knows what the plan is. Okay? So it would be best that she be supporting you with the plan. Because, if she doesn't know that this is a plan, then she's going to think, oh, well, maybe I'd better do something, or whatever. So, if she's going to do anything, she could help you to deal with how difficult it—it could be for you—listening to this going on. So do you think you could do that? That—you could talk with your mother about—so that she understands that this is an experiment that we're doing?

Carmen: Oh, yeah.

Arnie: Okay. Good. And you can also ask—by the way, you could ask your mother for her observations. And maybe you could share hers, as well as yours, about what was happening.

Carmen: Okay.

Arnie: Part of the purpose, too, about not trying to calm her down, and part of what we're thinking here, is that she needs—as she gets older, as people get older—they need to learn more things about how to calm themselves. Okay? So, part of this is, it's giving her an opportunity to begin to learn some of those things. It's part of growing up.

Schedule another session?

We frequently leave the timing for another appointment up to the client, even though we make a homework assignment. In our experience, the homework assignment gives clients a new way to begin thinking about their situation. Even if clients don't follow through with homework, if they return, they frequently comment on how the homework gave them something to think about.

Monte: And we have no idea when this is going to happen again, because the last one was about a week ago. It could happen tonight. It could happen tomorrow. It could happen next week. Who knows? Maybe it could go two or three—do you think it could go three weeks before—?

Carmen: That's possible.

Monte: So we just really don't know how long until this would happen again. And it probably wouldn't be real helpful for us to meet again until after this has happened. Does that make sense to you?

Carmen: Yeah, it makes sense.
Monte: Because you wouldn't have this data that we would need.
Carmen: Yeah. That's the whole reason why we're here.
Monte: I'm wondering if maybe two times—maybe if you give us a call maybe after the second time it happens. Or you could just walk in. That could be two months from now, or it could be two weeks from now. It could be tomorrow.
Carmen: Exactly.
Arnie: And you could even invite your mother to come, if you wanted to.
Carmen: Yeah.
Carmen: Yeah. So—well, yeah, I can do that, so—
Monte: Okay. Great.
Arnie: Good.
Carmen: Nice meeting you.

(As we rise and shake hands, Arnie says to Julia, "You have a good handshake." She grins broadly as she walks out.)

Carmen wanted to know if this was a serious problem and wanted ideas about how to deal with crying episodes. This intervention was designed to address both of those wants. The idea of not intervening in the crying episodes had already been considered by Carmen. We gave her professional permission to do so, and she seemed prepared to carry out the experiment. We also addressed grandmother's unsuccessful attempts to help. This session was held in 2008. Carmen and Julia did not return for another session.

Conclusion

In this chapter we provided a description of the single-session mindset that is critical to walk-in work. We also discussed tenets and assumption that are foundational to walk-in practice as well as basic guidelines for conducting walk-in sessions.

Some clients will come for a walk-in session for their first experience with therapy. Others will come for a walk-in session following an earlier walk-in session that may have been days, months or years earlier. Still other clients may avail themselves of a walk-in session days, weeks, or years after a course of a more traditional series of multiple sessions. We have found that a single-session mindset has advantages over one that expects that clients will need or want multiple sessions.

The case example presented in this chapter is typical of the way we handle walk-in sessions. As we pointed out earlier, a walk-in service does not have the luxury of extensive screening ahead of a session. We never know what problems will come through the clinic door. We could just as easily have presented a case where marital infidelity, worries about suicide, or a chronic psychiatric patient's problems in living were the presenting issues. For the most part, the organization of the session would have been very similar to this one.

References

Amundson, Jon (1996). Why pragmatics is probably enough for now. *Family Process, 35*, 473-486.

Andersen, T. (1987). The reflecting team: Dialogue and meta-dialogue in clinical work. *Family Process, 26*, 415-428.

Berg, I.K. & Dolan, Y., (2001). *Tales of solutions: A collection of hope inspiring stories.* New York: W. W. Norton & Co.

Berg, I. K., & Miller, S. D., (1992). Working with the problem drinker: A solution focused approach. New York: Norton

Bobele, M., Lopez, S.S.-G., Scamardo, M., & Solórzano, B. (2008). Single-session walk-in therapy with Mexican-American clients. *Journal of Systemic Therapies,* 27, 75-89.

Boscolo, L., Cecchin, G., Hoffman, L., & Penn, P. (1987). *Milan systemic family therapy.* New York: Basic Books

Brown, J., Dreis, S., & Nace, D. K. (1999). What really makes a difference in psychotherapy outcome: Why does managed care want to know? In Hubble, Mark A., Duncan, Barry L., & Miller, Scott D. (Eds.). (1999). *The Heart and Soul of Change: What Works in Therapy.* Washington, DC: American Psychological Association.

de Shazer, Steve (1985). *Keys to solution in brief therapy.* New York: W W Norton & Co.

Duncan, B.L., and Miller, S.D. (2000). *The heroic client: Doing client-directed, outcome-informed therapy.* San Francisco: Jossey-Bass.

Duncan, B, Miller, S., Sparks, J., Claud, D., Reynold, L, Brown, J., & Johnson, L. (2003). The Session rating scale: preliminary psychometric properties of a "working" alliance measure. *Journal of Brief Therapy, 3,* 3-12.

Fisch, R. *(1994). Basic elements in the brief therapies.* In M.F. Hoyt (Ed.), Constructive Therapies 1. New York: Guilford.

Freedman, J., & Combs, G. *(1996). Narrative therapy: The social construction of preferred realities.* New York: W. W. Norton & Co.

Haley, J. *(1973). Problem solving therapy. New York: Jossey-Bass.*

Haley, J, & Richeport-Haley, M. (2003). *The art of strategic therapy.* New York: Brunner-Routledge.

Houger Limacher, Lori (2003). *Commendations: The healing potential of one family systems nursing intervention.* (Unpublished doctoral thesis). Calgary, Alberta, Canada: University of Calgary.

Hubble, Mark A., Duncan, Barry L., & Miller, Scott D. (Eds.). (1999). *The heart and soul of change: What works in therapy.* Washington, DC: American Psychological Association.

Lawson, A., McElheran, N., & Slive, A. (1997). Single session walk-in therapy: A model for the 21st century. *Family Therapy News,* 30(4), 15-25.

Lawson, A., McElheran, N., & Slive, A. (2006). *Why clients return to a single session walk-in counselling service.* (Unpublished manuscript). Wood's Homes Eastside Family Centre, Calgary, Alberta, Canada.

Lipchick, E. (2002) *Beyond technique in solution-focused therapy.* New York: Guilford.

Madanes, C. (1981). *Strategic family therapy.* San Francisco: Jossey-Bass.

McElheran, N., & Harper-Jaques, S. (1994). Commendations: A resource intervention for clinical practice. *Clinical Nurse Specialist, 8*, 7-10.

O'Hanlon, W. & Weiner-Davis, M. (1989). *In search of solutions: A new direction in psychotherapy.* W. W. Norton & Company, Inc.: New York.

Prochaska, J. O. & C. C. DiClemente (1982). Transtheoretical therapy: Toward a more integrative model of change. *Psychotherapy: Theory, Research and Practice* 19, 276-288.

Ray, W. & Keeney, B. (1993). *Resource focused therapy.* London: Karnac.

Slive, A., MacLaurin, B., Oakander, M., & Amundson, J. (1995). Walk-in single sessions: A new paradigm in clinical service delivery. *Journal of Systemic Therapies,* 14, 3-11.

Slive, A., McElheran, N., & Lawson, A. (2001). Family therapy in walk-in mental health clinics. In M. MacFarlane (Ed.), *Family therapy and mental health: Innovations in theory and practice* (pp 261-285). New York: Haworth.

Slive, A., McElheran, N. & Lawson, A. (2008). How brief does it get? Walk-in single session therapy. *Journal of Systemic Therapies,* 27, 5-22.

Talmon, M. (1990). *Single-session therapy.* San Francisco: Jossey-Bass.

Walter, J. & Peller, J. (1992). *Becoming solution-focused in brief therapy.* New York: Taylor & Francis.

Wampold, B. E., (2001). *The great psychotherapy debate: Models, methods and findings.* Mahwah N.J: Lawrence Erlbaum Associates, Publishers.

Watzlawick, Paul, Weakland, John H. & Fisch, Richard (1988). *Change: Principles of problem formation and problem resolution.* New York: W. W. Norton.

Weakland, J., Segal, L. & Fisch, R. (1982). *The tactics of change.* San Francisco: Jossey-Bass.

White, M. (1986). Negative explanation, restraint and double description: A template for family therapy. *Family Process, 25*, 169-184.

White, M., and Epston, D., (1990). *Narrative means to therapeutic ends.* New York: W. W. Norton & Co.

Young, K. (2008). From waiting lists to walk-in: Stories from a walk-in therapy clinic. *Journal of Systemic Therapies,* 27, 23-39.

Chapter 4

Single-Session Stories

Compiled and Edited by

Kyle Green, MS

The following chapter is a collection of single-session case examples provided by current and former graduate counseling psychology students at Our Lady of the Lake University (OLLU) with various levels of experience. Some of these case examples were conducted at the Community Counseling Service (CCS) (Chapter 7). Others were conducted at off-campus practicum sites or in private practices. Typically, student therapists practice therapy and receive supervision exclusively at CCS for the first two semesters of the counseling psychology program. Master's and doctoral level therapists are then placed in off-campus sites to suppliment their continued training at CCS.

These eleven case examples illustrate students' work in a variety of mental health facilities, including hospitals, local nonprofit agencies, private practice, and community mental health clinics. Depending on the site, services are offered by appointment only, on a walk-in basis, or both. All of the case examples were conducted from a single-session mindset in which the therapist assumed that this session could be the first and last. This chapter emphasizes how Single-Session Therapy (SST) can be used with a variety of clients and a variety of presenting concerns. They are case examples with couples, individuals and families from diverse cultural heritages.

Some of the services were provided by individual therapists and some were provided by co-therapists. A few of the therapy sessions were supervised live. Some had team involvement while others did not. The names of clients have been changed to protect their identity. Moreover, some organizations requested that we withhold their names from publication; we have respected their wishes.

The Green Room

My name is Gaby Nuñez and I am currently in my second year of the Marriage and Family Therapy program at OLLU specializing in a certification to serve the mental health needs of the Latino population. I have interests in multiculturalism, systemic therapy and humanitarian work. I have worked with varied populations including: at-risk youths, individuals with HIV, sexually-abused children, adolescents and adults in the legal system, family conflict, and substance abuse. I have also worked in diverse settings: community mental health, hospitals, residential treatment centers, nonprofit organizations, and schools. In the future, I plan to earn a doctoral degree and work with human-trafficking victims.

A school counselor referred Christina, 32 years old, and her son Eddie, 8 years old, to the CCS. On the intake form, Christina stated that Eddie suffered from "anger management problems, ADHD, and had suicidal ideation." The intake form further read that Eddie had cut himself with a tape-dispenser at school and said that he no longer wanted to live. During the presession consultation, the team suggested possible ways to address the suicidal thoughts, get a clearer understanding of what Eddie's reasons were for saying he no longer wanted to live, and a plan for gathering more information about his homelife. The co-therapist and I were first-year master's students in our first semester working with clients. After reading the intake form, my co-therapist and I had imagined either a child running all over the room, bouncing off the walls and ignoring any type of re-direction, or the complete opposite, a quiet child who might need several sessions to get to know us and several more to allow us to explore his wish to no longer live.

When we actually started the session, Christina, an articulate and smiling woman, walked into the therapy room embracing her seemingly shy son, Eddie. We began by getting to know them and reviewing the consent information. We learned that Christina was a single mother of five children. Eddie listened carefully and rarely spoke. We interviewed for strengths in the family and recognized that Christina was very hard-working. She and her children valued bonding and helping each other. We also learned that Eddie was a good older brother who often helped to care for his younger brother with Down syndrome. When Christina was comfortable with us, she revealed that the school counselor was concerned about Eddie's possible suicidal ideation.

We asked Christina, "Are you worried about Eddie having suicidal thoughts?" Christina answered that the school counselor had made her worry, but that Eddie had told her that he did not intend to kill himself—that he had simply been angry. We followed up with "Are you worried that Eddie might actually do it?" Christina replied "no" and assured us that everything at home appeared to be problem free. When we then turned our attention to Eddie and asked if he knew what "Mommy" and we were talking about, he shook his head "no." We asked him if he remembered the tape dispenser incident and he replied "yes." We encouraged him to recount what had happened. He insisted that he had not wanted to kill himself.

It was at that point that we learned that Eddie had a speech impediment, which often frustrated him when he could not express what he wanted. He explained that he had cut himself accidentally with the tape dispenser while he was working with the special education teacher. He also explained that he had been angry because another child had hit him. When he said aloud that he did not want to live, he had meant that he did not want to be there, in that particular room, at that time. Christina confirmed that Eddie had a learning disability and easily became angry when he became frustrated with his schoolwork.

We asked them to describe the anger in behavioral terms. Christina informed us that when Eddie got angry he yelled, threw tantrums, and sometimes cried. She added that Eddie rarely became angry at home but that he frequently became angry at school, often daily. We then asked about exceptions: "Are there other times when Eddie gets angry? How often does he get angry? What types of things does he do when he gets angry?" We discovered that Eddie only got angry when he was at school. Christina said that he missed his previous school where the teachers let him go to a "Green Room" so he could calm down. Eddie agreed and said that he wanted to be in the "Green Room" school. Christina added that she had recently transferred Eddie to a new school so that he could attend school with his younger brother. The new school had not yet implemented a behavioral plan for him like the one at his previous school. She added that she had not yet met with the teachers and the principal at the new school.

We then asked about what had helped Eddie calm down in the past, Christina restated that anger was not a problem for him at home. She also thought that the previous school's strategy of allowing him to walk out of class to the Green Room had been helpful. The Green Room gave him comfort, had padded walls, and enabled him to vent with his Special Education teacher.

At that point in the interview, we decided to take a consultation break and consult with the rest of the team. We asked Christina and Eddie, while we took the consultation, to brainstorm about other things that Eddie might possibly do to manage his anger.

After the break, we complimented Christina on how much importance she placed on her children's education. We told her the entire team was impressed with her ability to be very proactive and take care of all her demanding responsibilities. We also acknowledged Eddie's efforts to be a good older brother. We commended him on his ability to recognize when he was getting angry and needed to leave a situation. Christina was pleased to hear this and adamantly stated that she would move her son back to his old school and go back to the behavioral plan that was working, even if it meant she would have to drive out of her way to take him.

We were very surprised with her decision to switch Eddie back to his old school and agreed that it would be worth trying again. Christina thanked us. We then asked her if she would like to come back to tell us how Eddie did with his familiar routine at his previous school. Christina agreed to set up an appointment for the following week to tell us how things went for her family. The following week, she cancelled and rescheduled an appointment for the week after that. Christina cancelled that session. She said that her family no longer needed services. Christina added that she would call to schedule an appointment if they needed counseling services in the future.

Some therapists may speculate that Christina and Eddie did not return to therapy because they did not get what they needed. I venture to say otherwise. Christina had a clear goal for therapy and got what she came for: a solution to her son's problem at school. Rather than going through behavior modification techniques, or running through endless lists of possible ways for Eddie to cope with frustration and anger, we maximized the potential for therapy in one session. We narrowed the database, empathized with the family's situation, and looked for strengths and resources. Lastly, we looked for solutions, including ones that had worked in the past, and empowered the family to try them. Perhaps she would not have scheduled a second appointment if we had worded the question differently while giving her options to reschedule at a later date or walk-in at a time of her choosing.

"I Want to Live My Normal Life Again"

My name is Karissa Gilmore. I am a second year doctoral student in the Counseling Psychology program at OLLU. I have had a wide range of clinical experiences providing services to children, families, couples, and adults. My training has prepared me to be culturally competent and given me the knowledge to be able to work with clients who have diverse mental health diagnoses.

Currently, I am working towards licensure as a Licensed Professional Counselor in Texas. I am also a part-time counselor at the Rape Crisis Center (RCC) in San Antonio where I have over two years' experience working with trauma and sexual abuse survivors. I have provided services to children and teenagers at the center, incorporating play and art into the therapy.

Alison was a sophomore college student native to San Antonio from a large Hispanic family that was supportive and actively involved in her life. Alison was an only child but had cousins who were "like brothers and sisters." Alison lived at home with her parents, was working at a part-time job, and held an officer's position in an honor society at her college.

In my experience working at the RCC, I found that a brief therapy approach that focused on solutions and was future-oriented was often what clients needed. Such an approach enabled clients to move forward and was preferable to re-telling unhelpful, discouraging stories from the past. I approached this session from a Solution-Focused Therapy stance, which, in the end, was the right fit for Alison.

Alison decided to make an appointment for counseling because she was "stuck and unsure of what to do." She explained that she had just ended a relationship with her boyfriend who had sexually abused her. Alison said that she was confused by her conflicting thoughts. She still desired to be with her boyfriend even though he had hurt her several times in the past.

Alison came to her counseling session knowing exactly what changes she wanted to make in her life: "I just want to live my normal life again without him in it. I want to stop crying all of the time." This goal was quickly identified, with little effort on my part. In order to refine this into a well-formed therapeutic goal, I asked Alison about small specific examples of what she would be doing differently in her life if the problem were gone, and she was not crying as much. "Normal" and "balance" were two reoccurring words Alison used to describe her life once the desired changes occurred. We refined what her "normal" life would look like, and what she would be doing when she had "balance." Alison gave clear answers to these questions that included examples such as going to her aerobics class twice a week, taking at least twenty minutes in the morning to polish her nails or put on make-up, and going to lunch more often with her friends and family.

As we talked about her life as a student, the conversation turned to identifying present exceptions to her complaint—things that she was already doing to address her presenting issues. With little guidance from me, she spontaneously described exceptions that were already occurring at her work and through her involvement with school. In the previous week, she went out with friends for dinner and had a great time talking and meeting new people.

At the end of the session, I complimented Alison on her strong sense of self-awareness. I thought it was very important for me to acknowledge the loss of the relationship and how much it was still hurting her. I told her that it was obvious she knew what she wanted out of life and what made her happy. I also explained to Alison that it was understandable for her to grieve the loss of her two-year relationship. She had trusted her boyfriend to love her and care for her. He had betrayed that trust by sexually abusing her. I said I understood how such a betrayal could be hurtful.

For homework, I asked Alison not to change anything, yet. I supported her need to take the time and energy to grieve the relationship before making any further changes. I encouraged her to find time to allow herself to continue grieve. Further, I asked her to write down the things she was doing that she wanted to take with her in her new normal life.

This session was not a planned single-session case. Initially, I was under the impression that Alison would be returning, because we scheduled an appointment for the next week. Before that appointment, she called and asked to reschedule for the next week. Alison did not arrive for the second rescheduled appointment. When I called her to follow up, I learned that she "did not feel a need to come back to therapy for now." Alison explained that she was able to do the homework task that she was assigned at the end of our session. By doing the assignment, Alison said that she, "realized all of the things that she was already doing" without her boyfriend in her life. Alison had already begun moving forward and doing the things she wanted to without realizing it. The homework assignment had helped her take stock of the progress she had already made, on her own. It should be noted that this pattern of scheduling and canceling appointments is a relatively common occurrence in many mental health agencies.

I think this session resulted in a single-session because Alison was able to identify a goal, recognize several times when parts of that goal were already happening and give herself permission to cry over someone who hurt her. I used questions to find exceptions and provided an atmosphere of empathic listening and understanding. This helped Alison take hold of the resources and strengths that she had within and around her. When she was able to take a step back, Alison recognized her own abilities and resilience.

0.5 is better than 0.0

Presenting concerns and session summary

My name is Laurel Bluntzer and I am a first year doctoral student in the Counseling Psychology program at OLLU. While earning my master's degree in Counseling Psychology, I worked with individuals, couples, and families in both inpatient and outpatient settings. I am particularly interested in couples and family therapy, women's issues, and alternative behavioral strategies for coping and stress reduction. I also currently work with individuals who are living with chronic pain and their families. My therapeutic approach is strength -based, utilizing Solution-Focused and Narrative theoretical orientations. My co-therapist and I saw the following case at the CCS.

Angela was a Caucasian in her early twenties. She and her stepmother, Mary, made an appointment at the CCS for therapy after Angela made a serious suicide attempt three days before our session. My co-therapist, also a master's student at OLLU, saw Angela and Mary. Angela had been hospitalized for the attempted suicide. She, with the help of her stepmother, explained that she would like to be able to cope with everyday stress more effectively. She identified the main stressors in her life as: a recent breakup with her girlfriend, financial concerns, physical distance from her son, her mother's upcoming release from prison (because she thought that she would have to care for her mother), and the pressure she felt from her father's expectations.

Laurel: Tell us how we can be helpful to you today. *(This is a common single-session question designed to understand what the client wants from the therapy session today.)*

Angela: I don't know; I was told to come here. That's exactly why I'm here.

Laurel: Okay, so who told you to come?

Angela: Baptist Hospital.

Laurel: And so they said it would be a good idea for you to call and make an appointment?

Angela: Well they gave me a timeline and told me I had to seek counseling and told me I had to do so many things or they were going to try and put me in Laurel Ridge (a psychiatric hospital), and I was not going to go to Laurel Ridge so I did exactly what they said. But if you're wondering why I was at Baptist Hospital it is because I tried to OD and commit suicide and...

Laurel: And that wasn't too long ago, right?

Angela: Three days ago.

Angela then told us that she has seen her family physician, Dr. Martinez since the time of the suicide attempt. Angela described Dr. Martinez as someone who cared for her and someone she trusted. We sought to gain an idea about what Dr. Martinez would notice about Angela if she began to solve the problem that brought her to our session. Only three days after a suicide attempt, Angela was finding it difficult in the session to identify what she would like to be different in her life. However, by asking about Dr. Martinez's perspective, Angela was able to imagine what could be different in her life. With these questions we attempted to arrive at a goal for therapy.

Angela: I saw him (Dr. Martinez) yesterday because I had 24 hours to see him.

Laurel: Did you guys talk about anything or did he offer you any advice that was helpful to you?

Angela: He told me he agreed with what they (the staff at the hospital) said… that I need to seek counseling because it's probably got a lot to do with what goes on in my day-to-day life, which he has seen my mom, seen my family, and he knows more about all the ins and outs and he said that it would probably be good to follow through with it.

Laurel: Is he someone that you trust—you trust his personal opinion?

Angela: Oh yeah, I would do anything he tells me to do—just about.

Laurel: Yeah so he cares about you a lot?

Angela: Yes he's been my personal doctor for eight years.

Laurel: What do you think that Dr. Martinez would say that we should focus on or talk about in our session together since he knows you pretty well? What do you think he would like to see? *(This question was strategically designed to gain an outside perspective and move the client to a well-formed goal.)*

Mary: He would like to see her be able to cope with everyday stress levels, you know, learn how to talk to people.

Angela: He says I need to develop life skills, that I don't know how to handle like, that I over stress, that I over worry.

Mary: Well you do, but a lot of it you bring on yourself and you worry about it for no reason. You shouldn't—it's something you shouldn't worry about.

Laurel: *(asking Angela about Mary's statement)* Okay, so do you agree with her assessments?

Angela: Yeah.

Mary: I've been through a lot of things, like she has and I've just learned to cope with them a little better than she knows how to, but I think when she gets my age, she'll be alright.

Use of scaling questions for goal setting

Laurel: So, if you were to think about your ability to cope with stress, before, when you were in school, when you were working at Pizza Hut, um on a scale from 1 (not very much ability to cope with stress) to 10 (you deal with stress perfectly fine) where were you when all of that was going on?

Angela: Maybe like a two.

Laurel: Like a two? Okay, so back then you were at a two. Where are you today?

Angela: Right now any little thing would probably set me off, so I mean it's probably at zero.

Laurel: Well I think that, I just have to say that with your mom getting out of prison, and your trips to see your son, I can understand how you would be experiencing a really, really difficult time. I would be surprised if you were just happy as could be because there are a lot of things going on. You are at a zero today. If you walked out of here and were miraculously at a 0.5, what would be different, what would you be doing? What would you be able to do that you can't do now? *(This was a question designed to focus on small change. Small changes lead to bigger changes (Walter & Peller, 1992).*

Angela: There are a lot of things I can't do now. I can't handle sitting down and actually discussing anything with anybody right now without yelling.

Laurel: Is that something that you might be able to do if you were at a 0.5?

Angela: I don't talk to anybody about anything and maybe that's part of the reason what led me as far as I went. The most people I talk to is her (pointing to her stepmother), and my ex-girlfriend.

Mary: Yeah but you hadn't talked to me in like four days except for little things.

Laurel: Okay, would that be a sign that you were maybe at a 0.5 or nearing a 1 if you started talking to her (Mary) again a little bit here and there?

Mary: I think it has helped her. She's doing a little better today than she was last night. Do you agree?

Angela: *(Nods)*

Laurel: So how were you able to do a little bit better today? What are you doing that's different? *(This was a question designed to emphasize a client's strengths and ability to create positive change. It can also encourage a client to do more of what was working.)*

Angela: Because I vented last night.

Laurel: Okay, so that's helping you a little bit.

Laurel: Is talking more, expressing your feelings more, is that something that you want, or not really?

Angela: I want to be able to do it, but I want to be able to do it with everybody.

After we felt that we had a clear goal, we took a break to consult with our team. We returned to the session with commendations for Angela and Mary. We then asked her to notice times, in the coming days, when she feels herself coping slightly better, at a 0.5 on the scale. We also asked Mary to notice times when she observes Angela coping slightly better. Angela then identified some behaviors that might help her to cope better, such as writing and taking a bath.

Commendations

Laurel: We really want to thank both of you for coming in today, I know this is kind of impromptu for you, Mary, but it helps us to have another perspective, so we appreciate you making the long drive through the rain. I think that it is obvious to us and the team that the two of you have a pretty special relationship. I think that just sitting here and talking to you for an hour, that's apparent, and we are so glad that you are here for Angela and that she has you to go to.

Um, Angela we have seen that you have really followed through with what the hospital has asked you to do, you have taken Dr. Martinez's concerns to heart and come to see us. But we also know that you are here for you, ultimately, and for what you want to work on and we know that you have goals and things you want to change. So we are definitely glad you are here. But we also want to work on what you want to work on. And you guys both have a lot of good ideas about what those things are. You want to cope better with everyday life stresses and with some not so everyday life stresses like your mom coming out of prison, the expectations that your dad has for you, and talking to people in general, and I know you have a hard time with that but you've done a stunning job here today talking with us.

Bridge

Laurel: Angela you said that you were at a 0 today in your ability to cope with stress but we know that at one time you were at a 2, so there must have been some things that you were doing when you were at a 2 that were helping you to cope with stress a little bit more…

Homework

Laurel: What we want you to do over the next week or so is we want you to notice times when you are able to cope a little bit better, just a 0.5 and when you realize, okay I'm coping a little bit better… it's not good… it's not where I want to be, but it's a little bit better. We want you to look around and say, "what am I doing, what's helping me, who's around me, what's going on that's helping me to cope a little bit better." We want you to write it down...

Laurel *(to Mary):* And what we want you to do is to be on the sidelines and just notice, I know you already do… you are our eyes and ears, and you can tell us, on this day she was coping a little bit better and I noticed she was doing this differently or I noticed she did this for herself. Does that sound like something you can do?

Mary *(to Angela):* You can do that. You write anyway.

Angela: That's the only way I feel like I can express myself.

Laurel: So if over the next week you are feeling pretty stressed out and you start writing….. that's the perfect example of something…you might take a bath or whatever it is.

Angela: I do that too.

This session was not a planned single-session, but we specifically asked the client if she felt it would be helpful to schedule another appointment so as not to assume that Angela needed another session. At the time of this session, Angela indicated that she would like to return for a second appointment. However, during a follow-up call, Angela reported that she had made improvements and felt as though she was coping better. Angela expressed satisfaction with the services that she received during her single-session. She seemed to feel as though she was headed toward a solution through improved coping.

Sometimes Fear is Normal

My name is Samantha Anders and I am a fourth year doctoral student in the Counseling Psychology program at OLLU. I have worked in the counseling field for 12 years and have experience working with adults in drug and alcohol rehabilitation, at-risk youth, and family therapy. I recently completed a practicum placement at the Cancer Therapy & Research Center (CTRC) in San Antonio. I am currently completing a practicum in Texana in Richmond, Texas performing psychological assessments with individuals with intellectual and developmental disabilities. The CTRC is a multidisciplinary, comprehensive cancer treatment center. Physicians and other professionals (psychologists, social workers, nutritionists) come together in one central location to treat patients as a team in disease-specific multidisciplinary clinics. CTRC offers a full spectrum of clinical and support services to meet the medical, nutritional, emotional and spiritual needs of the patient, from diagnosis through treatment, rehabilitation, discharge and follow-up care. CTRC provides two doctoral practicum placements per year for OLLU PsyD students.

Debbie was a 36 year-old Caucasian patient, who had previously been treated by Dr. Marcus at the CTRC. She had recently finished chemotherapy for breast cancer and was in full remission. Debbie was diagnosed with breast cancer in January 2010 and began receiving chemotherapy and radiation treatments at CTRC. During her treatment Debbie met with Dr. Marcus on various occasions to discuss psychosocial stressors that were impeding her treatment, including financial and marital difficulties. She found therapy helpful in these situations, and in May 2010 stated she did not feel further treatment was necessary. She showed improvement on her National Comprehensive Cancer Network (NCCN) Distress Management Measure and Beck Depression Inventory-Fast Screen (BDI-FS) for Medical Patients that supported her statements of improvement. In June 2010 Debbie was informed her breast cancer was in full remission. She was scheduled for a yearly follow-up with her oncologist at CTRC and terminated therapy.

Debbie called Dr. Marcus' office in August 2010 with concerns over recently increased anxiety and fear of relapse. Dr. Marcus referred Debbie to me. Her referral information indicated she wanted to "check-in," and she scheduled an appointment. From the referral it was not clear how many sessions Debbie had in mind. However, within the first ten minutes it became clear she did not wish to re-engage regular therapy sessions but preferred to get a handle on the current situation. My questions were aimed at understanding what events had prompted her phone call, what presession changes might have occurred (Weiner-Davis, deShazer, & Gingrich, 1987), and exploring exceptions to her worries about a relapse, because she had previously been able to competently manage very stressful situations.

We discussed the treatment course for breast cancer and the ways in which it is physically and mentally debilitating. We discussed relapse rates, developed a "what if" plan and practiced relaxation techniques. During the session it appeared that Debbie primarily wanted reassurance that she was not crazy for being fearful of relapse. She shared that her husband often told her "Just don't think about it," and she found this frustrating and anxiety provoking. We discussed the coping mechanisms she already had in place—walking and yoga—to manage her anxiety, and discussed how she might incorporate these into her routine once or twice more per week. At the end of the session Debbie stated that she felt much more relaxed and felt sure she had a strong plan to deal with her anxiety. Debbie and I discussed possible future sessions and she stated she did not feel a future session was necessary at this time though she would call if she needed.

After this session I had no further contact with Debbie, although future sessions remained a possibility. For Debbie, the single-session approach was helpful because it allowed her to focus on the current problem that was causing disruption in her life. The fear of relapse is a normal response for someone who has completed cancer treatment. Debbie acknowledged her fear and attempted to solve the problem but her attempts had failed and she felt stuck. In general, Debbie felt her life was on track and did not warrant further explanation. Her goal for this session was to troubleshoot the one place where she felt stuck. By normalizing her fears, staying focused on the present, exploring exceptions, and developing a list of positive behaviors she could use in place of her anxious behaviors, Debbie was able to feel more in control of her fear.

It's Not a Symptom - It's a Protective Strategy

My name is Shawne Ortiz and I am a fourth year doctoral student in the Counseling Psychology program at OLLU. As a licensed professional counselor in Texas and a Nationally Certified Counselor, I have worked in a variety of settings including community mental health, private practice, residential treatment, and hospitals, with a wide range of clients. I have over seven years' experience providing psychotherapy primarily with individuals, families, children, and couples who are experiencing a number of mental health diagnoses.

Mark was an 8 year-old African American accompanied by his father and paternal grandmother. He and his family were seen at the Center for Miracles at Christus Santa Rosa Children's Hospital in downtown San Antonio. Anthony Nguyen and I were co-therapists for this family. Anthony was also a fourth year doctoral student in the Counseling Psychology program. The Center for Miracles was created in 2006 in response to the number of child deaths resulting from severe abuse and neglect that occurred in the San Antonio area. The Center is a clinic comprised of doctors, nurses, social workers, and psychotherapists who provide a multidisciplinary team approach to evaluating severe cases of child abuse and neglect. The clients who are seen at the Center for Miracles are on an appointment-only basis at the request of Child Protective Services (CPS) or law enforcement.

This family was involved with CPS because Mark's biological mother had allegedly abused him. In the most recent incident, Mark's mother hit him with her car while he was riding his bike in the street in front of their home. Neighbors witnessed the incident and called the police. The father and grandmother described Mark's mother as very abusive. Neighbors reported she would lock him out of the house for hours at a time. Mark's grandmother added that Mark's mother would hit him on his head and face.

By the time they arrived for counseling, CPS had placed Mark with his father. His grandmother said she was worried that he was traumatized and would have trouble adjusting. His father said Mark had been with him for a few weeks at that time and was doing well in his new school. He said Mark was very well mannered and would answer "Yes, ma'am," "Yes sir," etc. He also remarked that Mark was very helpful around the house. For example, he made his bed before school and cleaned up after himself. Mark's father had no complaints about his son's behavior. Mark's grandmother's fear was that he had been traumatized because, in the past, he had wiped feces on his bedroom wall in his mother's home. She wanted to know why someone would do that.

To help Mark's grandmother and father gain a different perspective on Mark's behavior, we shared with her a story about a client of a colleague. In that case, a young boy was wiping feces on himself and the walls in the foster home where he was living. The youngster was being bullied and abused by older boys in the home, so, when he wiped feces on himself or the walls, the other kids left him alone. When I explained to her that this other boy had used this as a way to defend himself from being abused, it made sense to her. It explained why her own grandson may have done this in the past. When reframed as a protective strategy, and an effective one at that, it made perfect sense to her and she no longer viewed her grandson's behavior as abnormal. Rather it seemed a smart way to protect himself from his mother.

During the session it became apparent that Mark was not displaying disruptive or disturbing behavior in his father's care. The family viewed the counseling appointment as preventative, much like a check up with their family doctor. We discussed how children are much more resilient than adults and how the idea of feeling safe could be enough for Mark to cope with everything he has gone through.

We encouraged the family to continue being supportive of Mark. We stated that, if there were changes in his behavior, they could return to counseling at anytime. They seemed to need the reassurance from us that Mark was okay for them to see him as doing well. After discussion of Mark's past behavior I asked what we could focus on that would be helpful concerning Mark's current behavior. They could not name anything that was currently of concern. That is when it became apparent the session would be a single-session.

When we asked more about behaviors that would indicate Mark was having trouble adjusting, no one offered any signs that would indicate he was having problems. Mark said that he was doing well and liked being at his father's home. The grandmother said that she felt he was doing well but wanted to continue to see a counselor as a check-up to make sure he was okay. They scheduled another appointment "just in case," but were informed if they did not need it they could cancel. They did not show up for the scheduled appointment and when I contacted the father, he said Mark was doing well and did not need further counseling.

This was a case in which it was apparent early on that the child was not suffering any apparent psychological discomfort: he was doing well in school and at home. During this session, Anthony and I utilized a strength-based approach to emphasize the many positive behaviors that Mark was demonstrating in his new home. We emphasized how the compassion and love shown by Mark's father and paternal grandmother could be enough to let Mark know he was in a safe place. We also utilized questions that emphasized Mark's positive coping skills and how he was an example of the resilience of children in overcoming traumatic experiences. Both Mark's father and paternal grandmother were able to recognize that Mark was not displaying disturbing behavior that would indicate he was in distress. With the strength-based questions, we were able to get the family to focus on what was currently going well. Moreover, by telling the family they could cancel the next appointment if they did not need it we created a positive vision of the future in which Mark would adjust just fine. This reassured Mark's father and grandmother that Mark was normal.

A Time to Celebrate

My name is Tanya M. Rugen and I am currently employed at the Baptist Child Family Service working towards state licensure. I received my master's degree in Counseling Psychology from OLLU in 2009. I have had the privilege of working with an array of client populations. I've worked from a solution-focused approach with marginalized homeless individuals, the mentally ill, adolescents in the juvenile justice system, and people with everyday problems. Currently, I work systemically as a Circle of Support Facilitator at CCS with children, adolescents, their families, and probation/parole staff involved in the juvenile justice system as the young people make the transition back into the community. Consulting with these diverse populations has been very rewarding to me, as I have utilized my theory in evoking hopefulness and directing clients towards recovery and transformation.

Perry was a 42 year-old Caucasian student, and twenty-year employee at a local gas station. He walked into the CCS in April of 2009. This was the second time Perry had utilized our walk-in service. My co-therapist and I were master's level graduate students with approximately two years of counseling experience.

Perry's presenting concern was that in the previous week his boss "implied that he was lazy." When we asked him how we could be helpful that day, he responded that he was irritated and had to get things off his chest. In addition, he needed someone to talk to. When we asked what he wanted to get out of the counseling session, he said his goal was to be able to let go of his boss's opinion. Further, he explained that he wanted his job performance to please himself, not his boss. He added that he had to make things at work less personal. We asked Perry to assess his hope of letting go of his boss's opinion. He said he was at a 5 on a 10-point scale, and that he knew he would be letting go if he felt he was at a "comfortable standpoint."

We worked collaboratively with a team of master's level students and supervisors via closed circuit television. An intercom allowed them to call into the therapy room to make suggestions throughout the session. The team called to ask Perry how much time he thought it would take him to let go of his boss's opinion. He replied that he wasn't sure but, had already begun to feel better that morning knowing he was coming into therapy and having had a few days off from his workplace. The therapists understood this occurrence as pre-session change (Weiner-Davis, deShazer, & Gingrich, 1987), change that the client had made before walking into the clinic.

He then commented on the upcoming one-year anniversary of his stroke. He stated, "I have come to the realization that life is too short to waste on people's opinions like my boss's." He pointed out that he was able to drive better, had stopped pacing, was doing well in school, and had taken a stand with his girlfriend. We amplified his progress at work, school, and relationships, such as writing a ten page paper, giving a presentation in school, and knowing that overreacting to his boss's opinion by acting out in a negative way could cause his boss to fire him.

After a break for a consultation with the team, we relayed that the team had noticed how insightful he was. We commended him for his mature perspective about life, good decision making skills, ability to re-evaluate priorities in his life, and his self-validation. We emphasized self-validation because he had wanted the validation of his therapists in his earlier walk-in session. He was also commended for his ability to decide when to take advantage of the walk-in service. For homework we asked him to celebrate the anniversary of his stroke. By assigning this task, the therapists wanted Perry to celebrate his ongoing recovery and comfort. Perry stated, "I have been thinking about doing that by maybe taking donuts to the hospital where I was cared for."

The therapists and team treated this as a single session by amplifying his solution talk of presession change, utilizing the hopefulness scale, and commending his realization that life is too short to waste on other people's opinions. Importantly, the one-year anniversary of Perry's stroke was highlighted as a significant event. At the end of the session he stated, "I almost died; therefore my anniversary is a milestone; I am almost normal; I might even be normal." At the end of the session, Perry told us that he felt better, and that he would return to the walk-in clinic if needed.

She Was Already Doing It

My name is Mary Sichi and I am a third year doctoral student in Counseling Psychology at OLLU, with 2 years of doctoral-level practicum experience at the CCS. I also have a master's degree in Clinical Psychology from St. Mary's University in San Antonio, Texas. In my work at the CCS and at previous practicum sites, including an in-patient unit of the state hospital, I have worked with clients from diverse backgrounds, dealing with a variety of difficulties. I am interested in how individuals and families find unique ways to cope with the challenges they encounter in their lives. My co-therapist was working on his master's degree and had one year of counseling experience.

Janice was a 34-year old married Latina who scheduled an appointment for therapy at the CCS in June of 2009. She was tall, energetic and straight-forward in her speech. Janice suffered from intense shoulder and knee pain resulting from an injury that occurred at work the previous year. She reported to us that she had always been a very independent person. She was unhappy with her current situation, because her recent surgery had left her dependent on others, especially her husband. Her injuries had limited her ability to work full-time and caused her pain in her current part-time position as a custodian. In spite of the sometimes crippling pain and multiple surgeries she described, Janice came across as a strong woman with a powerful physical presence in the room.

Janice stated that her goal in coming to therapy was to "feel like her old self again," or as she had felt before to her injury. She also said that she wanted to stop taking her frustration out on her husband. Janice talked about her lack of energy, her affinity for her godchildren, and her wishes to ameliorate the relationship with her husband. She had recently gone back on her antidepressant medication to help regulate her moods. When asked what she would be doing if she felt like her "old self again," Janice replied that she would be up at 6AM every day to take a walk. She reported that on those mornings in the past when she had been able to get up early and be active, her mood and frustration levels were usually improved for the rest of the day.

Utilizing the research of Sharry, Madden, Darmody, and Miller (2001), we made use of the consultation break time by having Janice complete a brief task while we consulted with the team. Before leaving the room, we asked her to write down some specific actions she could take to help her get up early in the morning, take a walk, and continue her day productively.

During the consultation break, members of the team observed that Janice had already taken steps to better her situation, such as scheduling an appointment for therapy and going back on her medication. As a team, we also discussed what we saw to be Janice's strengths; her previous independence and her current positive attitude coupled with a strong motivation to change. We agreed that the best way to help her would be to reflect to her our observation of these assets and to encourage her with our opinion that she was already well on her way toward achieving her goal.

When we returned, we found that Janice had completed her assignment by writing down a number of ideas, some of which she shared with us. She listed going to bed early the night before, talking to her husband about her plans, and making coffee soon after getting up in the morning. We conveyed to Janice the team's observation that she had already taken significant steps to improve her situation. We also reflected on the positive elements and resources in her life, including her love for her godchildren and her supportive husband. For homework, we asked Janice to try out her idea about getting up early and to call the CCS every day and leave a message for us indicating how her morning had gone.

When we offered a second appointment, Janice assured us that although she had found the session helpful, she would call to schedule another appointment if she felt that she needed to come back. She did not call in to report her daily progress or respond to a message left for her, nor did she call to schedule a second appointment.

This case was not planned as a single-session and unfortunately, we were unable to contact Janice for a follow-up interview. However, her strengths and previously high level of functioning made it likely that she got what she needed from this one session in order to continue the psychological recovery that she had already begun.

Because we were working from a brief therapy model, we asked questions designed to focus on Janice's current strengths in an effort to highlight steps that she was already taking towards recovery. For example, by asking Janice what currently gave her joy in her life, we found out that she enjoyed spending time with her godchildren, and that this was a significant motivator for her to overcome her pain so she could again engage in activities with them. We were interested in helping Janice articulate specific, behaviorally-defined goals. We asked questions such as, "If you were feeling back to your old self, what would you be doing?" and "What would your husband notice you doing differently if you were back to your old self?" These questions helped Janice to formulate the simple but physically and psychologically beneficial goal of getting up and taking a walk every morning.

As Janice stated, she was not comfortable relying on others for help, and I think that our session confirmed her characteristic belief that she was best able to create and enact her own solutions. The intervention, perhaps intrusive in its requirement that she check in daily, was designed to facilitate the realization that she did not need the kind of help she might receive from a long-term therapy relationship and thereby highlighted the strengths she already possessed. Based on these intended effects of the intervention and on the personal strength and energy she displayed within the therapy session, it seemed like that Janice did not schedule a second appointment because she decided that she was not the kind of person who needed ongoing therapy.

Not Like My Mother

My name is Shannon Stovall and I am a third year doctoral student in the Counseling Psychology program at OLLU. As a licensed professional counselor in Texas, I have practiced in several settings, including the CCS, a partial hospitalization program, a family violence center, a Head Start center, the Job Corps, and private practice. At this time, I am also one of four full-time clinical therapists in a local psychiatric partial hospitalization program. I am also teaching an undergraduate Introductory Psychology course.

Ann and her grandmother, Linda, came for one family therapy session at the CCS. Ashley and I, both first year doctoral students at the time, saw them together. Ann, a 15-year-old Latina, had been living with her grandmother, a 54-year old Latina, for about four years. Ann reported that she asked her grandmother to make an appointment, because she wanted to "keep from being like mom." According to Ann and Linda, Ann's mother, Sandra, was in and out of their lives, struggled with drug abuse, and engaged in many intimate relationships. Linda recalled that Sandra began "doing drugs" and "being promiscuous" when she was fourteen years old. Linda told us she was concerned about Ann and did not want her to become like Sandra. Linda had already seen signs that Ann was making some of the same poor choices. Linda gave two examples of poor decision making: Ann recently slept with her boyfriend for the first time, and she was experimenting with marijuana. Linda was concerned that these were signs that Ann was going to be like her mother and become more reckless in her choices.

Ann quietly listened during the first few minutes of the session as her grandmother told us about these concerns. Ann then told us that she loved her grandmother and wanted to continue sharing everything with her. Linda said that this was one of the differences between Ann and Sandra, because Sandra never shared anything.

Ashley and I explored this further and asked about how each of them helped to create this sharing atmosphere. Ann was able to say that she shared with her grandmother because she knew her grandmother loved her and would take care of her. We asked Ann what she thought about her grandmother's concerns. Ann agreed that she did not want to become like her mother nor make poor choices. Further, Ann said she needed to continue to avoid making negative choices and increase making better ones.

I asked her about "better choices" she had already started making. Ann said one example was participating in more physical activities; she enjoyed working out and dancing. These activities motivated her to stay healthy. Ann also pointed out that she decided to come for counseling and she was trying to argue less at home. Ashley asked Ann how she might continue making these better choices. Ann recognized one thing that would help her continue to make better choices would be interacting with a more positive peer group. She explained that her boyfriend and several of the girls she dances with are positive people in her life. Ann also revealed that she would like to be a United States Marine some day. She acknowledged that in order to achieve that goal, she needed to stop smoking marijuana, focus on her grades, and avoid becoming pregnant at fifteen like her mother.

When we asked Ann about the first small goal that we could focus on in that session, Ann offered that she would like to start thinking about her actions before she did them. We followed up on this to gain clarity and encourage Ann to voice her own plan for this goal. Ann elaborated that if she thought about her actions first, she could write down a "pro and con list," or at least make one in her head. We asked her how many pros and cons she would need to list before deciding on a choice. She laughed and told us just one for each if they were big enough, but maybe three or four on most things. Linda reminded us about their concern with drug abuse and asked whether Ann could make a pros and cons list about drugs during the session. Ann laughed and told her grandmother "I'm not stupid. I know it's bad. I don't know the pros about doing it, except that it relaxes me and my friends do it."

Following up on her statement, we asked, "So, it sounds like you have a few pros on the list. What would be the cons?" Ann responded by saying, "It could keep me from being an officer if I get caught or have a criminal record. And, it's bad for you." Linda interjected that it had also been a gateway drug for Ann's mother. After we reviewed with Ann the steps involved in making a pro and con list, she told us that she planned to do more of those in the future because she was "smart enough to keep on track and be a better person than my mom."

Furthermore, Ann and Linda wanted to be able to maintain open communication so that each felt supported by the other. Ann reported that when the appointment had been made, she was at a 1 on a scale of how "on track" she was (1 being "not at all" and 10 being "right on track). Linda also reported she thought Ann was about a 1 the previous week when the appointment was made. In the session, Ann stated she now felt she was at a 7, because she had made positive changes over the past week to work toward being on track. These changes included staying away from bad influences and talking more to her grandmother about her life. Linda thought that Ann was a 5 on being on track, because she was cautious about the change being so new. When we asked about how she might move to a 6 on the scale, Linda stated that "just having Ann keep talking to me" would make her more confident about change.

Ashley and I went back to consult with our team. During this intersession break, the team members commented that the homework should be something both Ann and Linda would be able to engage in together. The team also voiced the idea, based on session observations, that Linda and Ann's session might be a single-session case. Our supervisor encouraged us to ask them when they would like to reschedule and let them set the timeframe. That would allow them to decide whether they wanted another appointment or not.

When we returned, we commended Linda and Ann for the mutual love and respect for each other that they had demonstrated. We told them that we recognized how difficult it was to maintain the open communication and trust they enjoyed with one another. Ann was recognized for her good judgment and her motivation to make a better life for herself. As a homework assignment over the next few weeks, we asked Ann to consider additional "positive activities" she could engage in that replace the time that she used to spend with her "negative peer group." We encouraged her to pick activities that she thought would help her stay "on track" with making better choices.

When we asked Ann and Linda when they would like to schedule another appointment, they both hesitated and said that they would like an appointment for two weeks later. During the postsession, our supervisor reflected that the clients might have felt that setting another appointment was expected. She suggested in the future we might ask first if these clients would like to come back, before asking when. As a team we predicted that these clients would not come back in for the second session, because this session identified multiple strengths, highlighted the successes they already achieved, and through the homework, promoted ways they would be able to continue this change on their own. Two weeks later, when we called to confirm the appointment, Linda cancelled, as we had predicted. She reported that things were going very well for them both. She and Ann had discussed the upcoming appointment and decided it was not needed. She added that if, in the future, they needed to come back in and talk, she would keep the number and both therapists' names handy. She thanked us again for the help we provided.

Brian and Tammy: Single-Session Therapy

My name is Kyle Green and I am a fourth year doctoral student in the Counseling Psychology program at OLLU. I have provided counseling and assessment services in a variety of settings around the San Antonio area, including hospitals, residential treatment facilities, and community agencies. I have received training in multicultural competence and have had the opportunity to work with a wide variety of culturally diverse individuals, couples, and families. I was either the co-therapist or the individual counselor on the following three single-session case examples.

Brian (32-years old) and Tammy (23-years old) were a high school educated Caucasian couple who have been married for approximately two years. Tammy scheduled an appointment with the CCS because the couple had been arguing frequently. The couple had moved to the San Antonio area approximately one year earlier when his employer transferred Brian. They were both born and raised in Florida, where all their friends and family lived. Brian was a skilled laborer and Tammy was a stay-at-home mother. The couple's first child was born three months earlier.

The therapy team decided that the two co-therapists who would conduct the session would consist of one male and one female graduate student therapist. Both of us were doctoral students with two years of direct therapy experience. We conceptualized the case using Solution-Focused Therapy (SFT). The team approach (Palazzoli, Boscolo, Cecchin, & Prata, 1978) was explained to the couple and they consented to therapy.

The couple explained that they came to the CCS because they had been experiencing marital difficulties associated with being new parents and with being separated from their family and friends. The couple was also financially stressed because Brian's work (construction) was seasonal, and this was the idle period of the year. In his free time, Brian had been spending a substantial amount of time playing video games and going to a local bar with his co-workers. This angered Tammy because it left her home alone raising their three month-old infant when she needed Brian's support. Brian's complaint was that Tammy was smothering him and not allowing him to "be a man."

During the session, we listened to the couple's presenting concerns and normalized the challenges that came with becoming new parents and being separated from a support system. We made a point to listen and validate each of the partner's concerns so that each of them felt heard and respected. We also took this stance so that the couple would not feel that the therapists were taking sides with either partner. This approach afforded the team therapeutic maneuverability within the session and helped to establish a therapeutic alliance.

As is common with the SFT approach, we identified the strengths and resources that the couple brought to the therapy session. The couple explained that there was a considerable amount of love in the relationship and that they were 100% committed to each other. Tammy appreciated Brian's sense of humor and Brian loved how Tammy was "always there for him." During the team consultation, the team identified numerous accommodations and collaboratively developed a summation message for the couple. After the team consultation, we complimented the couple and gave them a "homework assignment" to gain a more thorough understanding of the couple's relationship. The team assigned the formula first session task which asked the couple to notice the things that are going right in their life and that they would not like therapy to change (de Shazer, 1985). The couple agreed to complete the assignment and scheduled another therapy appointment for the following week. The couple seemed enthusiastic about the task and reported looking forward to our next meeting.

The couple returned to the clinic the following week. There was a noticeable change in their appearance and attitude. They were smiling and speaking in a very respectful way towards and about each other. Brian and Tammy had completed their version of the homework assignment and produced a list of things they loved about each other. This was not the precise assignment that we had asked them to complete, but we sensed the couple's positive change in attitude, so we did not interrupt. Each partner proceeded to read their list aloud and elaborated on how they could use these attributes to compromise with each other. Items that topped Brian's list were that Tammy was a great mother, he liked how she took care of the house, and she was a very passionate person. Tammy's list, which she wrote down, included Brian's hard work ethic, he was a talented chef, he never judged her, and he unconditionally loved her. Both lists stated that the couple loved each other so much that they could always make up after an argument. It became apparent that the couple was not using this session to address their presenting marital concerns from one week ago. Rather, they were celebrating their successful completion of the assignment and reporting that they had received what they had desired from therapy. The couple was congratulated for their efforts and reminded that CCS would be available to them should the need for counseling services arise in the future. Therapy was terminated.

This is a good example of a non-planned single session of therapy. The team approached the session from a strength-based orientation and helped the couple identify their own solutions to their concerns. The therapists asked questions relating to positive coping and problem resolution strategies that the couple had successfully employed in the past as opposed to focusing on the relationship deficits. One strength-based strategy that we utilized during the first and second session was to scale the couple from 0-10 on a communication scale with 10 meaning the best communication possible and 0 meaning the opposite. During the first session Brian and Tammy each stated a 5. During the second session, Brian stated he was a 7 and Tammy stated she was an 8. We then asked each partner what they did to move up on the communication scale. Brian stated that he told himself to remain calm and thought about the consequences if he over-reacted when the couple had emotional conversations. Tammy stated that she began to communicate more directly as opposed to dropping hints, which is what she had done in the past. She mentioned that Brian did not always pick up on the hints and Brian agreed. Brian and Tammy each identified strategies that they were employing to improve communication instead of focusing on the problems that brought them to therapy.

The therapy session could have taken a much different path if the therapists chose to discuss Tammy's perception that Brian was being irresponsible or selfish or Brian's perception that Tammy was treating him like a child. In this instance, the SFT approach to marital therapy was a good fit for the couple, and one session was all that was necessary for them to achieve their therapy goal. It should be noted that we viewed this as a single-session case even though the couple came to the clinic twice, because the second session was used by the couple to emphasize their success in meeting their therapy goal and to terminate therapy. The couple got everything they needed from the first session.

Recognizing Her Strengths and Accomplishments

Yolanda was a 30 year old Latina single parent raising two children ages 8 and 4. Both children had been previously diagnosed with autism. Yolanda's husband, Ricardo, died unexpectedly approximately 6 months earlier owing to gang related violence. Since that time, she had been working two jobs to support her children. Yolanda's mother, Patrice, was the only person helping her with childcare responsibilities.

Yolanda made an appointment with Any Baby Can (ABC) because she felt stressed and overwhelmed with raising her children. ABC is a non-profit organization that serves children with disabilities and their families. ABC and OLLU have a partnership to provide free counseling services to ABC clients. The counseling services provided are identical to the team approach discussed in earlier case examples, with one licensed psychologist supervisor and four training therapists. My co-therapist and I (Kyle Green) were graduate students from OLLU. My co-therapist was a master's level student with one year of direct client experience.

Yolanda described her daily routine of waking up early, getting her children ready for school, going to work, and picking up her children late in the evening from her mother's house. She stated that she was stressed from working six to seven days a week, being a single parent with limited social support, and getting very little sleep. She also stated that she hasn't had the time to "properly" grieve the loss of her husband.

The team conceptualized Yolanda's case using SFT. After listening to Yolanda's problem description, the team collaboratively identified Yolanda's treatment goal. Yolanda wanted to be a "soccer mom" to her children. We invited Yolanda to describe what she meant by "soccer mom" in concrete, observable terms in an attempt to uncover a well-formed goal (Berg & Miller, 1992; Walter & Peller, 1992). She explained that a soccer mom does not yell and is well prepared. As we further examined her responses, she explained that a soccer mom would complete laundry, lay out the children's next day's clothing, and prepare breakfast and school lunches in the evening prior to the next school day. She would also get the children to the school bus stop on time. We used the Solution-Focused technique of scaling questions to solidify her treatment goal (Walter & Peller, 1992). Yolanda was currently a 4 on a scale with 10 meaning a complete soccer mom and 0 meaning the opposite. Yolanda identified the 0 as being a "crazy person." We utilized this scale and the client's language to help identify exceptions—examples of times when Yolanda was already being the soccer mom.

Yolanda returned for a second session the next week. We used another 10 -point scale to ask Yolanda to assess whether therapy had been successful and if she would not need to attend any longer. This time she estimated 7. She stated that, in the preceding week, she had brought the children to the school bus stop on time on three occasions. She also acknowledged that she did not yell at home every day. When we asked if there were other instances also, she sat quietly for a few moments and then, with a surprised expression, said that there were. "On Thursday, I laid the kids clothes out the night before, fed them before bath time, and made their breakfast before going to sleep. I did not need to yell all day because I was prepared and organized. That day was a 7."

We complimented her and emphasized her accomplishments. Yolanda expressed relief that she was already accomplishing her goal for treatment and is the occasional "soccer mom." The team and Yolanda mutually agreed to schedule a return appointment in one week, but Yolanda did not return for her appointment the following week. I made a follow-up phone call and she assured us that she got what she needed from therapy and did not need to return at that time. She stated that she would like to return in the future to work on her grief over the loss of her husband. I encouraged her to return whenever she felt the need.

In this example, the team used SFT to identify Yolanda's strengths. In the process of using strength based questioning, Yolanda recognized that she was successfully raising her children. She was able to identify times in which she was the mother she wanted to be and was able to identify how she was doing it. She left the therapy session with a plan in mind to continue her success.

It should also be noted that even though the client scheduled a subsequent therapy appointment, we were working from a single-session mindset. We believed that positive change can occur from a single session of therapy, but we also believed that clients know what is best for them. We routinely offer every client additional therapy sessions if they think that additional sessions might be helpful. Taking a cue from Possibilities Therapy, I prefer to end sessions by asking clients if they would like to schedule another appointment or if they had received what they needed from therapy during the present session (O'Hanlon, 1998). Many clients respond by saying that their therapy goals were met and one session was all they needed.

Living Life to the Fullest

Mr. Martinez was a 65 year-old Latino diagnosed with terminal cancer. He was seen at a large government health care organization in San Antonio, Texas that specializes in healthcare for U.S. armed forces veterans. I (Kyle Green) was his assigned therapist and worked with him from a Solution-Focused perspective. It should be noted that I worked with Mr. Martinez alone and did not have the luxury of a therapy team or co-therapist described in earlier cases in this chapter.

Mr. Martinez's physicians estimated that he had roughly six months to live and was referred for mental health services to help him cope with his recent diagnosis and prognosis. He had bone cancer that was especially pronounced in his hips and left leg. He required the use of a walker to assist him into the clinic. When I met with Mr. Martinez, he moved and spoke very slowly. He appeared depressed, and emotionless.

He had been married for over thirty years and had two adult daughters living nearby. He was an active person prior to his diagnosis, was very spiritual, and considered his family to be the most important thing in his life. His recent lack of mobility "severely" affected him because he had been active, motivated, and energetic. Mr. Martinez recalled that he used to be very active in his church and coached several youth sports programs.

When I asked what he would like to get out of coming to therapy, Mr. Martinez looked confused and stated "I don't know." Then I asked him a common single-session therapy first question: "If our time here today were successful, what would be different in your life?" He stated that he had been neglecting his family and his responsibilities for some time due to his illness and depressed mood. If our session were successful, Mr. Martinez said that he would begin living the way he had before receiving his diagnosis. I explored this idea a little further.

He stated that he was a church elder and had recently been "skipping" church and Bible study. He had also been neglecting his household chores and the management of his six acre plot of land outside the San Antonio area. Finally, he stated that he had been neglecting his family, choosing to isolate himself in his room. He added that he missed his two daughters and would like to repair a strained relationship with his brother.

I reflected that it sounded as if he was a very spiritual person and that his family was very important to him. He agreed and went on to explain how much he loved his family and how proud he was of his two daughters. I invited Mr. Martinez to explain how his spirituality and family has helped him through this difficult time. He explained that his wife had been his sole caretaker and had been an "absolute angel." He said that his two daughters were raised very well, were college educated, chose to continue to live near the family, and represented the family in a very respectful way. Lastly, he stated that even though he had missed church recently, he continually looked to his faith for guidance.

Mr. Martinez began speaking at a normal rate and sat up in his chair when he began identifying his strengths. It was apparent that his support system was very active and influential to him. I reflected this back to him and he agreed.

Nearing the end of the session, I invited Mr. Martinez to identify what was next for him. This is a future oriented question that implies hope. He came up with numerous tasks that he wanted to achieve. He wanted to clean out his workshop behind his house, complete his taxes, begin attending church on Sundays and bible study one evening a week, and clean up the brush that had accumulated on his land. I inquired if this was possible or realistic due to his current health condition, and he mentioned that he could do the taxes and hire someone to take care of his workshop and plot of land (with his supervision of course). This brief therapy question allowed Mr. Martinez to identify his strengths, amplify his resilience, and buy into to his goal setting. This is also a good example of clients having the strength and resources necessary to solve their problems. Because I asked questions instead of making suggestions, Mr. Martinez was able to identify a number of solutions that I never would have recommended. This speaks to how clients know what is best for them.

I complimented Mr. Martinez on raising such a respectful family and having such a good attitude despite his potentially terminal diagnosis. I then asked "did you think you would be in this place (mood) after an hour?" He replied that this was the last thing that he thought could happen and this was the "kick in the ass" he needed. He made an appointment in one month to give him time to complete all of his self-assigned tasks.

Mr. Martinez returned in one month and his physical condition had worsened. He required the use of a wheel chair at that point, but still had an amazing attitude. He discussed his accomplishments and even reported that his story was the topic of discussion at the Bible study class. He reported that his story helped other people and that he had accepted that he was ready for "his God to take him whenever." He had made amends with his brother and he planned to continue helping others as long as he could. This was his new mission. He had accomplished about half of the tasks assigned at the previous visit, and was still motivated to accomplish them.

This case really speaks volumes to how resilient and strong people can be. Approaching this case using SFT amplified Mr. Martinez's strengths and achievements. Despite his potentially terminal illness, he was able to identify healthy coping strategies and a positive support system. We consider this case to be a single-session even though the client returned in one month, because he was able to identify and set a plan in place to achieve his treatment goals in only one session. Sometimes one session is all a client needs.

References

Berg, I. K., & Miller, S. D. (1992). *Working with the problem-drinker: A solution focused approach.* New York: Norton.

de Shazer, S. (1985). *Keys to solution in brief therapy.* New York: Norton.

O'Hanlon, B. (1998). Possibility therapy: An inclusive, collaborative, solution-based model of psychotherapy. In Hoyt, M. F. (Ed.), *The Handbook of Constructive Therapies* (pp. 137-158). San Francisco: Jossey-Bass Inc.

Palazzoli, M. S., Boscolo, L., Cecchin, G., & Prata, G. (1978). *Paradox and counterparadox.* New York: Aronson.

Sharry, J., Madden, B., Darmody, M., & Miller, S. D. (2001). Giving our clients the break: Applications of client-directed outcome-informed clinical work. *The Journal of Systemic Therapies,* 20(3), 68-76.

Walter, J. & Peller, J. (1992). *Becoming solution-focused in brief therapy.* New York: Brunner/Mazel.

Weiner-Davis, M., deShazer, S., & Gingrich, W. J. (1987). Building on pretreatment change to construct the therapeutic solution: An exploratory study. *Journal of Marital and Family Therapy,* 13, 359-363.

Part Two
Walk-In Counseling in Varying Locations

Chapter 5

Walk-In Counseling Center: Minneapolis, Minnesota

Gary Richard Schoener

It was in the early months of 1969 that Dr. Alan Sroufe, a professor at the University of Minnesota in the Department of Child Development, called a meeting in order to form a Minnesota Chapter of Psychologists for Social Action at the University of Minnesota. As the mixture of students, university-based professionals, and psychologists from the community discussed possible projects, it was suggested that one project be "a free clinic." The free clinic movement had begun a few years earlier with the creation of the Haight Ashbury Free Clinic in San Francisco. Dr. David Smith's book *Love Needs Care* (1971) provides an excellent overview of the beginnings of this movement, and a national perspective can be found in *The Free Clinic: A Community Approach to Health Care and Drug Abuse* (Smith et. al., 1971).

Several months earlier, in the fall of 1968 a group of pediatricians established the TeenAge Medical Service (TAMS) in a house in south Minneapolis. Its focus was on providing services to young people, some of whom were runaways, many who were quite alienated.

One of the psychologists present at the Minnesota organizing meeting, Dr. Marian Hall, had been involved with TAMS and suggested that we join those pediatricians and offer counseling services. In May of 1969 a group of psychologist volunteers began offering free counseling to those who came to TAMS for medical services. The original staffing involved a mixture of graduate students, professors, and community-based mental health professionals.

The name *Walk-In Counseling Center* was locally unique and chosen to reflect the fact that, unlike other outpatient counseling centers, this one did not require an appointment. It was also chosen because it was neutral—being a somewhat projective test in that potential clients could see in it anything they chose.

The Context

Numerous agencies sprung up simultaneously in the early 70s. Just as Walk In began providing services, a hotline called Youth Emergency Services also started providing phone counseling services to young people—especially runaways who were facing issues of abuse. Some graduate students, including myself, volunteered in both services. Youth Emergency Service evolved to serve people of all ages and today is called Crisis Connection. At about the same time, two nuns, Sisters Marlene Barghini and Rita Steinhagen, created our state's first runaway house, The Bridge for Runaways, which has continued through the present.

Within the first year of Walk-In's opening its doors, fledgling drug abuse related treatment programs began to appear in our local community. Initially they focused on helping young people deal with marijuana and especially with hallucinogens. "Talk downs" of people having "bad trips" were a major undertaking. Within a few years these programs began dealing with young people who were having troubles with habitual drug use—first amphetamines, then a variety of prescription drugs, and eventually heroin.

At the time it was not lawful to provide health care services to minors without parental consent, but for the most part the police looked the other way. In the few encounters our staff had with law enforcement, individual officers and some precinct captains made it clear that the police were glad someone was reaching out to help these young people. It was not until 1972 that legislation was passed allowing minors to access and consent to services on their own.

The evolution of the early youth crisis services, including walk-in counseling centers, was happening around the United States, and the Subcommittee on Children and Youth of the Senate Committee on Labor and Public Welfare, chaired by Senator Birch Bayh, held hearings on youth crisis services in Minneapolis in 1972 (Schoener, 1972). Although it was labeled by one youth leader as "the participation put-on," meaning an attempt to co-opt young people (Moffet, 1971), the Nixon administration had a genuine concern about reaching out to disaffected young people. An Office of Youth and Student Affairs (OYSA) collected information on alternative youth services and eventually arranged for direct consultation to Elliott Richardson, the Secretary of HEW. As a result of Walk-In's pioneering work, I was one of the people who provided consultation to the Secretary, OYSA, and also the Special Action Office on Drug Abuse Prevention in the White House and the Drug Abuse Section of the U.S. Office of Education.

Early Challenges

Preparing volunteers to deal with alienated young people was an immediate challenge for the Walk-In Counseling Center. Volunteers were first challenged to learn about street drugs and their abuse. This was followed by ten sexuality when young people came in to discuss sexual relationships, concerns about pregnancy, and decisions regarding birth control and eventually abortion.

When TAMS moved to the house next door and only Walk-In remained in the original house, the age span of walk-in clients began to broaden. Along with this came a greater variety of clients. Among them were gays and lesbians who came in depressed due to having had a relationship break up. At that time there was a drop-in center called *Gay House,* where some counseling was done, but there were no real counseling services serving the gay and lesbian population. *Walk-In* pioneered providing couples counseling for gay couples. Soon we helped a small group of openly gay and lesbian counselors to set up a program that became *Gay and Lesbian Community Services.* Walk-In also provided consultation to a group seeking to amend the Minneapolis Civil Rights Ordinance to include sexual orientation issues. Further, Walk-in helped craft the ordinance that protected gay people from discrimination. The term "gay" was written into the law and was defined as "affectional or sexual preference," a definition that has been widely adopted.

Volunteers Need Coordination

For its first two years, Walk-In depended on donated space and the coordination of volunteers by other volunteers. By 1971, the Walk-In Board of Directors decided that there was going to be an ongoing need for the Center and that it was time to plan for paid staff. Walk-In and TeenAge Medical Service, submitted a grant request to the Governor's Crime Commission, our state's method of dispensing funds from the newly created Law Enforcement Assistance Administration. These funds were to be aimed at serving "potentially delinquent youth" and they provided key money for the early youth services. Soon Walk-In had a full time Executive Director, an Office

Coordinator, and a half time Community Coordinator. In 1973 when the state grant ran out, Hennepin County began providing community mental health funding. This funding was to continue for thirty years. The community mental health center movement was focused on outreach and service access, and Walk-In was ready-made for that task. By this time the Center had added a Clinic Director and a Director of Consultation & Training Services to its staff.

The Payment for Services

Because the Center was largely staffed by volunteers, fees were not charged. The Center's services remain free today. Volunteers donate their time in order that at least one service in the community can operate without entry barriers (including fees). The Hennepin County Medical Center had a Crisis Intervention Center that did not charge those who came in crisis from about 1971 to 1991, but otherwise service access everywhere did require payment or insurance. Over this same period of time most of the original "free clinics" began to charge fees and collect Medicaid and insurance payments as they evolved into community health clinics. Walk-In is unique, at least locally, in remaining "free"—fees are still not charged.

The Use of Volunteers

Because volunteer professionals have always done our primary clinical work, we have had a considerable focus on the recruitment and screening of volunteers. Throughout most of our history, recruitment was done via word of mouth with volunteers often recruiting each other. More recently the center has placed advertisements in professional publications had has developed a more active solicitation process. Our website at www.walkin.org is a part of this plan. Walk-In has always had a large number of volunteer counselors, but the recruitment of supervisors currently requires special effort. Those professionals must be experienced in psychology or clinical social work or a related field and also have supervisory experience.

The screening of volunteer applicants is rigorous. Those seeking to volunteer must fill out an application that is eight pages long. Prospective volunteers must provide reference information from at least two persons who have supervised their clinical work. Applicants must reveal any history of professional complaints or discipline. Moreover, they authorize Walk-In to speak with anyone, including but not limited to their references, to review their work history, skills, and ethical qualifications.

Each year approximately 125 professionals donate time as counselors and supervisors, and another 25 or so paraprofessionals volunteer as receptionists. Many of the receptionists are undergraduates who are considering going into a mental health field. Each quarter we have 11 or 12 teams consisting of a receptionist, a supervisor, and four or five counselors. Some volunteers have been with us for more than 30 years, others for only a year or two. Some begin as receptionists and come back as counselors; a few have become supervisors.

Volunteers have access to a small library of practice-related books supplemented by a relatively large library of training audiotapes and videotapes. We have job boards and notice boards for continuing education workshops. Periodically, volunteers are provided with memos regarding professional issues such as changes in child abuse reporting statutes, the duty to warn or protect, and other practice challenges. Some of this is made available on our website (www.walkin.org).

Some volunteers form long-term friendships or collegial relationships, and there have been a few successful marriages between volunteers. The opportunity to network with other professionals of diverse backgrounds is one of the lures of the center. When surveyed, Walk-In's volunteers have indicated that the ability to help others in the community and to get additional training and experience are the main reasons they donated their time. The key to the former lies in our supervision model.

The Supervision Model

In the early 1970's, our first director visited the Los Angeles Free Clinic. As a result of that visit, Walk-In decided to shift to a team supervision model. With this model counselors work on a team with a designated supervisor. Afternoon teams arrive at around noon and provide counseling from 1PM to 3 PM, and typically leave by 5 PM. Evening teams assemble by 6 PM, counsel from 6:30 to about 9 PM, and then have a team meeting. The supervisor oversees how clients are assigned and runs a case conference at the end of the clinic hours. In order to be available for quick consultations, the supervisor sees clients only if all the counselors are already occupied. Counselors who have questions about how to handle a situation or referral can, with the client's permission, excuse themselves to get consultation from either another counselor or the supervisor. In some situations a second therapist is invited into a session for co-therapy.

An interesting situation arose during a site visit by a team from the American Psychiatric Association (Glasscote et. al., 1995). The study required that someone from the accreditation team sit in on a session, but Walk-In had never allowed observers. However, we offered to put two of the visiting psychiatrists through our screening process, on the spot, so that they could become temporary team members. Both were exceptional professionals and they easily "passed" the screening. One of the sessions involved a client with a problem that was outside the experience of the walk-in counselor, but well within the visiting psychiatrist's expertise. With the client's and therapist's permission, he waded in and took over the session. The client received excellent service, and the regular counselor and the team benefited from some extraordinary unexpected training.

Walk-In developed a supervisory training program in the mid-1980s that involves a series of classes and readings followed by a stint as an assistant supervisor of a team. The supervisor is a team leader whose job it is to organize and oversee the team's efforts. The supervisor signs the contact forms in order to ensure that all cases are discussed. Supervisors vary as to how they conduct their team meetings, but Walk-In rules require that they have the last word in situations deemed by them to be life threatening to the client or third parties. Under those circumstances they can direct the counselors to take certain action. Otherwise, their focus is to provide feedback to counselors (and the supervisor) regarding any cases seen. The supervisor may also suggest and/or provide additional individual supervision of a case during clinic or at another time.

The paid staff—the Clinic Director and the Executive Director—are available for any additional consultation or to settle any disagreements or disputes. The Clinic & Administrative Coordinator and the Clinic Director solicit feedback during each quarter as to team functioning and the performance of counselors and supervisors. In 2010, periodic Saturday morning meetings of supervisors were begun as a way of sharing concerns and solutions about the challenges of team supervision.

Clients

In 2009 1,588 clients were seen for 5,231 counseling sessions. Forty-one percent had family incomes less than $10,000 a year. They came to Walk-In from more than 200 referral sources. About half of our clients had no insurance coverage. Those who had coverage had limited access to providers, or had a long wait for an appointment. Many of their insurance plans had high co-pays and large deductibles. Fifty-one percent of clients were male, and 49% women—a ratio that has held for a great many years. Forty five percent were single. Thirty-six percent had children. In terms of age, 4% were less than 20 years old and 3% were over 61 years old. Forty-percent were in their 20s, 25% in their 30s, 18% in their 40s, and 10% in their 50s. The cultural/racial composition mirrored that in the local community: 69% Caucasian, 19% African American, 4% Chicano/Latino, 3% Asian/Pacific Islander, 1% American Indian, and 4% Other.

Presenting complaints varied widely. Only a small percentage of our clients are seriously and persistently mentally ill. The majority of clients, regardless of diagnosis, were experiencing a situational problem of some sort. Depression, anxiety, problems with anger, and relationship problems are common. Clients include refugees and immigrants, torture victims, veterans and their families, homeless people, LGBT individuals, and abuse victims. Over the years shifts have occurred in the demographics of our clients. Such shifts are often the result of the existence of an alternative service provider or the fact that another service has become less available or closed down entirely. The most dramatic example was the creation of a great many youth-serving organizations that now assist many of the young people who came to Walk-In in the early 1970's.

Case Example 1

The following case is an example from the late 1970s in which the full team played a significant role.

A young man came into the Center one evening and indicated that he was depressed and struggling with a feeling that he "did not belong." Apparently, eight years earlier he had experienced the painful break off of a relationship, had left the United States, and enlisted in a foreign military service. This was during the war in Vietnam, a time of great turmoil and social change in the states. He had recently returned from abroad and was living in his old neighborhood, but did not feel at home.

He did understand things he was reading and experiencing, and although he felt like he was "going crazy," the team decided that this was a case of culture shock. After several team members participated in interviewing him, the team discussed the situation. They decided that having "missed" a critical period in history he was disoriented. No member of the team had ever seen such a situation, nor had they imagined it, but the more they discussed it the more it seemed to be a reasonable explanation.

The man was desperate, and there were no obvious places to refer him. The team decided to have him continue at Walk-In. The treatment plan involved a series of weekly assignments that involved trips to the public library, among other things. He was given assignments that involved viewing videotapes and reading, systematically and chronologically, about what had happened while he was gone. Eventually he was guided to reconnect with acquaintances from long ago. After a period of about seven months the client said he felt "grounded" and was feeling neither angst nor disorientation. The only debate was whether team members had gained more than their client by this revisit to times gone by.

It would be hard to categorize the creative approach taken by the team with this man's problem, but these example illustrates the value of immediate team consultation. Their approach was not part of any common therapeutic approach or model. Nothing in graduate training prepared our counselors for such a challenge, but by working together creatively they came up with an effective response.

The Walk-In Counseling Center Model

Counselors and supervisors come to the Walk-In Counseling Center with a great diversity of training and experiences. We provide them with orientation, but not explicitly with training in our specific model. We hope and expect that both the orientation and their work as a team member instills in them our model. Our model team consists of the supervisor, the therapists, and the receptionist. The receptionist plays a key role in the delivery of services and is expected to sit in on team meetings and have input into case discussions.

Recently, the Care Quality Committee of our board of directors defined our service model as follows:

> A wide range of individuals comes in to *Walk-In* with a great variety of needs and situations. The most critical expectation by *Walk-In* of its receptionists and counselors is that the client, to the degree possible, feels welcomed, and feels heard. It is presumed that the counselor obtains consultation from team supervisor or other team member as needed during the clinical encounter. The following are the procedures followed when a client arrives at the Center:
>
> 1. The client is welcomed by receptionist, provided with client handout, and offered a beverage. The receptionist asks whether they have been to Walk-In previously. If so, the client's file is located. The team supervisor decides which counselor will see the client.
> 2. The counselor greets the client, and if there is a chart, at least glances at it. The counselor asks the client if he has any questions about the handout and answers any questions about the service, confidentiality, etc.
> 3. The counselor asks client what brings them in—what they are seeking and how they got to us.
>   a) If coming at the request of a third party, the expectations of others are examined (family member, probation officer, social services, employer, halfway house, etc.).
>   b) What the client expects/wants is discussed, with a preliminary determination as to service expectations. Typical expectations include:

- Information about a problem; or getting help, etc.
- Issues with another service provider; possible complaint
- Help through a crisis or lapse in care by another program
- Support and guidance in a crisis situation
- Assistance in helping another person—family, friend, or neighbor
- Direct help with a personal problem.

4. The counselor determines the level of urgency and whether the client is at risk to harm self or others. If needed, consultation from a peer or the supervisor is obtained. If there is a risk of danger to self, a suicide assessment is done. If the risk involves danger to others, an assessment of risk level is done.
5. If the client is in crisis, crisis intervention is undertaken with a determination what additional help is needed. This can involve (a) referral for evaluation for hospitalization; (b) referral for emergency housing, shelter; (c) referral for medication or other care; (d) scheduling of follow-up by Walk-In; and/or (e) development of safety plans for situations where harm could occur.
6. If an assessment is needed, possibly for a third party, the counselor determines whether this is something appropriate to Walk-In, or obtains sufficient information and appropriate releases to facilitate this:
   a) If clinical assessment is needed to determine if someone has a problem (e.g. for access to housing, to qualify for a service, to get a referral);
   b) If the assessment requires testing which can be done at Walk-In (MCMI-III, MMPI-2, Beck scales, Hopkins Scale);
   c) Typically, Walk-In does not do forensic assessments, with the exception of evaluations of torture survivors in connection with asylum petitions (in order to obtain asylum, beyond physical evidence that they have been tortured, refugees are required to have a psychological assessment which finds psychological problems such as PTSD resulting from the torture).
7. If the client is seeking counseling help for a problem, a treatment plan is developed for short-term intervention—goals for an intervention of less than 10 sessions.
   a) This may be the only intervention planned.
   b) This may be in conjunction with the client being referred for other services.
   c) This may be a stop-gap type of care for someone who is awaiting services at another agency or program, or whose care has been temporarily interrupted due to unavailability of other service provider.
8. If the client is returning for ongoing counseling at Walk-In, the treat-

ment model presumes:

a) Building enough insight about the problem for the client to be able to carry out whatever interventions or "homework" assignments are made.

b) The client is provided with recommendations and/or tools to use to address distress symptoms such as anxiety, depression, etc.

c) The client is provided with recommendations for other potential assistance such as medications, support groups, other types of counseling.

d) The client is provided with recommendations or direct assistance in fostering better communication with regard to a relationship dispute or problem.

9. While there is not a single treatment model, a cognitive-behavioral approach is the most likely one for most of the situations at Walk-In, especially given the focus on short-term care, and the reality that most clients come for just a few sessions. These includes short-term interventions for depression, anxiety and panic, and reduction of distress in situations where emotional breakdown is occurring. The treatment can also include de-escalation of anger in family violence situations and the development of safety plans.
10. Interventions may involve other people in the client's life. For example, the identification of the need to confront a family situation such as substance abuse, alcoholism, gambling, threats, etc. Interventions can also involve dispute resolution and problem solving agreements between people—roommates, family members, etc.
11. History taking and the collection of collateral information are done as needed to carry out the assessment or counseling functions. Releases are obtained as needed.
12. If longer term care or support is clinically indicated or requested by the client, there is a review of what referral resource might be appropriate. If the counselor is willing to provide such a service there is a discussion with the supervisor or team as to appropriateness for Walk-In, as well as which counselor would be suitable.
13. Each session ends with a clarification of the plan of action that has been determined in that session.

The major difference between this model and what most volunteers are familiar with is the assumption that people seek our help for a wide range of reasons and that providing direct counseling or therapy may not be our response. The counselor may be answering a mental health question, making a social services referral, or helping a client clarify a problem. So the first session is not a mental health intake evaluation.

Our experience with clients is similar to most other agencies. About fifty percent of clients are seen only once, and the bulk of the others are seen for 2 to 5 sessions. A very small percentage of clients are seen for ongoing care of ten sessions or more. About 60% receive referrals at some point in the counseling process—either for basic or supplemental services.

Evaluation as a Service

One of the most critical needs that Walk-In responds to is the request for an immediate evaluation or assessment. Sometimes this is a request by a county social services department. In other cases it is in connection with an asylum petition by a refugee who is a torture survivor.

Recently a need has arisen to provide a mental health diagnosis for homeless persons seeking housing through a program requiring a mental health diagnosis.

Case Example 2

A young Hispanic man had been living in his car and was seeking housing that required a mental health diagnosis. Every place he called to make an appointment for a diagnostic interview said it would take two months to get one. At Walk-In he was interviewed for an hour and found to be depressed. We also administered a BDI-2 which further confirmed a moderate depression. Therapy was begun for the depression, he was given a referral for longer-term care, and a letter was written on his behalf and faxed to the housing program. He had a room to stay in that evening.

In our local community, full psychological assessments, when one can afford them, are difficult to obtain within a month's time. We find that most referral questions can be settled with minimal testing and a clinical interview.

Other Contributions: The Consultation and Training Role

One of the original goals of Walk-In was to provide a vehicle through which psychologists and other mental health professionals could donate *pro bono* services to the community. Another was that, in addition to counseling services, we also provide community education and consultation and training. Thus, our early work with young drug abusers led us to develop memos for the community on topics such as dealing with chronic hotline callers and responding clinically to flashbacks from "bad trips" on hallucinogens. We also became involved in helping other groups design and implement new services aimed at drug abuse treatment and prevention.

Walk-In was often in a position to organize cross-disciplinary solutions to problems and to convene meetings of diverse groups. Examples of such efforts included:

- Creation of the Metropolitan Drug Assembly, a consortium of groups who were addressing drug abuse problems.
- Development of youth diversion programs that were police-community programs designed to serve troubled young people.
- Creation of a metro area Free Clinic Consortium, which over the years evolved into a community health organization.
- Creation of the Consortium on Battered Women, which helped focus community attention on family violence and was eventually absorbed into state government.
- Developing community awareness and collaboration in dealing with rape and sexual assault. Following a highly successful conference in 1974 major improvements occurred in collaboration between police, prosecutors, emergency rooms, social services, and victims groups.
- The development of the Council of Mental Health Programs in Hennepin County, which continues today and is currently coordinated by Walk-In in an effort to maintain system-wide communication in an era of scant resources.

A Unexpected Role: Dealing With Those Who Had Bad Experiences Elsewhere

The fact that Walk-In had professional counselors, but was not part of any larger system, made it a safe place for clients who had a bad experience elsewhere to seek help. The fact that they did not have to give their real name also contributed to a feeling of safety. From the day the Center opened, a subset of its clients came in with complaints about other service providers. In 1974 the first of what was to become a deluge of clients alleging sexual misconduct by a prior helper was assisted in making a complaint to the board that licensed physicians. In 1976 the Center began offering therapy groups for women who had been sexually exploited by therapists or clergy. This work led to major developments in terms of program innovation, training, consultation, and ultimately changes in Minnesota's statutes (Gartrell et. al., 1989; Gonsiorek, 1995; Jorgenson & Schoener, 1994, Schoener & Milgrom, 1986, Schoener et. al., 1989).

Looking Ahead

The Walk-In Counseling Center, like all non-profits, is facing many economic challenges. With government funding cuts the Center no longer receives any public funding. So private fundraising and foundation grants will be key to our survival. By the same token, attracting good volunteers and retaining them is an ongoing challenge. We are dealing with new generations of young professionals and need to understand what incentives will cause them to volunteer.

The Center is currently developing relationships with other community programs, which will involve the lending of volunteers who will provide services under our supervision in other locations. This was last done in the 1970's to aid free medical clinics that were not able to provide their own counseling services. In the last four decades, the Walk-In Counseling Center has helped stimulate the growth of many other needed services, has provided some unique training experiences for thousands of professionals, and has played a role in shaping public policy regarding service delivery.

References

Gartrell, N., Herman, J., Olarte, S., Feldstein, M., Localio, R., & Schoener, G. (1989). Sexual abuse of patients by therapists: Strategies for offender management and rehabilitation. In Miller, R.D. (Ed.). *Legal implications of hospital policies and practices.* pp. 55 - 66, San Francisco: Jossey-Bass.

Glasscote, R.M., Raybin, J.B., Reifler, C.B. & Kane, A.W. (1975). *The alternate services: Their role in mental health. A field study of free clinics, runaway houses, counseling centers and the like.* Washington, DC: American Psychiatric Assn.

Gonsiorek, J. (Ed.) (1995). *The breach of trust: Sexual exploitation by health care professionals and clergy*, pp. 3 - 17. Newbury, CA: Sage Publications.

Joint Commission on Accreditation of Healthcare Organizations (2002). Preventing sexual abuse of clients in behavioral health care settings. In JCAHO *How to Recognize Abuse and Neglect*, pp. 124-134, Oakbrook Terrace, IL: Joint Commission Resources.

Jorgenson, L. & Schoener, G. (1994). Regulation in the U.S.A. In Jehu, D. (Ed.). *Patients as victims: Sexual abuse in psychotherapy and counselling*, pp. 149 - 176. London, England: John Wiley & Sons Ltd.

Milgrom, J.H. (1992). *Boundaries in professional relationships: A training manual.* Minneapolis, MN: Walk-In Counseling Center.

Moffet, T. (1971). *The participation put-on.* New York: Delacort Press.

Schoener, G. (1972). Walk-In Counseling Services. Youth Crisis Services. Hearing before the Subcommittee on Children and Youth, Committee on Labor and Public Welfare, U.S. Senate, 92nd Congress. pp. 95-100.

Schoener, G.R. and Milgrom, J.H. (1986). A Walk-In Counseling Center approach to therapist sexual misconduct. In Burgess, A.W. & Hartman,

C.R. (Eds.) *Sexual exploitation of patients by health professionals*, pp. 152 - 162, New York: Praeger.

Schoener, G.R., Gonsiorek, J.C., Milgrom, J.H., Leupker, E.T., & Conroe, R. (1989). *Psychotherapists' sexual involvement with clients: Intervention and prevention.* Minneapolis, MN: Walk-In Counseling Center.

Smith, D.E. (1971). *Love needs care: A history of San Francisco's Haight-Ashbury Free Medical Clinic and its pioneer role in treating drug abuse problems.* Boston: Little, Brown & Co.

Smith, D.E. with Bental, D.J. & Schwartz, J.L. (Eds.) (1971). *The free clinic: A community approach to health care and drug abuse.* Beloit, WI: STASH Press.

Chapter 6

The Eastside Family Centre: 20 Years of Single-Session Walk-in Therapy

Where We Have Been and Where We Are Going

Ryan Clements MSW, RSW
Nancy McElheran RN MN, RMFT
Lee Hackney R. M.Sc., R.Psych
Harry Park MSW, RSW

Origins of the Work

The Wood's Homes Eastside Family Centre (EFC) was the first resource of its kind in Canada to provide a walk-in approach to the delivery of community-based mental health services. The Centre's walk-in service emerged in 1990 from discussions with local Calgary community and political leaders in response to a growing concern regarding the lack of social service infrastructure on the east side of the city. The idea of developing an immediately accessible and economically feasible service similar to the city's growing number of walk-in medical clinics began to take shape as a strategy to deal with an increased need for quality mental health services.

The Centre's original intention was to address local community needs as the community defined them. Wood's Homes' Chief Executive Officer and Board of Directors, along with the provincial authority for the delivery of mental health services, began to meet with key eastside Calgary community representatives and service providers. A task force developed the vision of a one-stop, multi-faceted, multi-partnered service linked to other resources in the community. Comprised of local police, school principals, business owners, service providers, community activists, and the local child-protection office, the task force was chaired by a local community member. After the EFC opended, several members of the task force became the first members of an ogoing advisory councel. This council shaped the EFC's services over its first half-dozen years of operation by emphasizing its community mandate, locating the Centre in a busy shopping mall, determining hours of operation that met the needs of the community, and naming it the Eastside Family Centre. The advisory council also helped to define the guiding principles of the Centre that included immediate, accessible and affordable mental health walk-in services. These principles laid the foundation of the Centre's efforts to create community ownership (Slive et al., 1995; Slive et al., 2001). The Centre was gradually funded through the provincial health and child protection/family services authorities, provincial grants, city-based funding, and fundraising efforts including community donations.

The result was a unique and seamless network of partnered community counseling and crisis services for clients that included, in addition to the walk-in counseling service, the Wood's Homes child and family mobile crisis team, a counseling service for men who perpetrate domestic violence (provided by the local women's emergency shelter), and a nonprofit family service agency. The local legal guidance agency agreed to provide on-site consultation to low income clients on a referral basis that created a useful option for certain clinical interventions where access to legal support and information was critical for clients. These ancillary services co-located in the Centre and integrated their service delivery to ease cross-referrals and mutual collaboration. Local immigrant service agencies and other community groups were invited to make use of the Centre's rooms to conduct meetings, facilitate clinical and other group activities, and to provide on-site child care for single-parent families so that they could use any of the on-site services. A variety of community-based mental health professionals responded to the invitation to volunteer their time at the walk-in service, thus enhancing the resource base and building upon the community approach of the Centre.

To maintain this community driven philosophy, EFC staff worked alongside the advisory group to promote the Centre's services to local family physicians, schools and key community resource centres through a series of face-to-face meetings. Linkages with the area's hospital emergency and mental health systems were created and then enhanced by recruiting psychiatrists who agreed to provide consultation at the EFC four days per week. The EFC then offered training in the walk-in model to psychiatric residents and family practice interns (Slive et al., 2001; Slive et al., 2008). While beginning by adhering to the original vision of the eastside community, after 20 years the EFC now provides services to clients from across the city of Calgary. Supported by longstanding community relationships, the ongoing development of new partnerships and a reputation for high quality services, the Centre continues to grow (Miller & Slive, 2004). The EFC is now nationally accredited by Accreditation Canada (Canada's national accreditation body for medical services) and is recognized as a leader both in service delivery and in the training and development of professionals. An average of 8-10 graduate level students per year add to the Centre's clinical services through the provision of extended practicum internships.

The EFC provides approximately 2200 sessions each year to 3000 clients. Clients are referred to the Centre by a variety of sources. Twenty-five percent of clients hear about the Centre through word of mouth (friends, relatives, co-workers who have accessed the service), 18% are referred through the local health authority (hospitals, mental health clinics) as a part of treatment planning, 16% of clients are referred by their community school, 14% of clients are referred by their family physician or local walk-in medical clinic, while 10% of clients hear about the Centre via other community services.

Of the clients who present at the EFC annually, roughly 50% attend a single-session of therapy and do not require a referral for additional services, while 25% are referred to community-based mental health agencies, and 10% are referred to the provincial health care system's outpatient mental health resources or their family doctor. Less than 1% of all clients are referred to more intensive services such as hospital emergency or child protection services due to risk of harm to self, others, or a child. A note of interest is that 35% of the clients each year have been to the EFC on at least one previous occasion.

Theoretical Model

The EFC's theoretical model for the walk-in service, as articulated by Slive et al. (2008), was developed through eighteen years of practice experience, teaching and clinical supervision. The underpinnings of the model integrate current thinking regarding common factors in effective therapy (Hubble, Duncan & Miller, 1999; Duncan & Miller, 2000; Wampold, 2001), research on brief ıches (Bloom, 2001), and the work by Talmon and his associates le-session therapy. The model encapsulates theoretical features of tmodern, social constructionist, solution-focused and narrative approaches (Hoyt, 1994, 1996, 1998; White & Epston, 1990; Lipchik, 2002) and has been consistent over time with the view that no one therapeutic model or approach will fit every client. The EFC's interest is in finding out what will be useful for the client now and then "giving it to them" (Slive et al., 2001).

Consistent with this model is the belief that clients are in charge of the therapy and that each session is a consultation designed to move them in their desired direction. The model is heavily influenced by the structure of the service itself; it is a whole therapy, delivered in one hour, which invites a pragmatic approach to the clients' presenting concerns. The therapist encourages the clients to describe their problem in current terms and create specific goals to address them (Amundson, 1996). This service structure is based on the assumption that clients are the best judges of what they need and when they need it, and that the clients' resources and competencies can be mobilized to assist them in moving toward solving their problems.

The session format is guided by the work of the Milan group (Boscolo et al., 1987) and consists of five parts: the presession, interview, intersession, intervention and postsession debriefing. One-way mirrors and multidisciplinary therapy teams are used to facilitate this process. In the interview, therapeutic questions are designed to bring forth the following: the immediate contextual factors that lead the client to seek therapy now, the client's beliefs about the problem, and the smallest change that could be useful to them in their current situation (Slive et al., 2001, 2008). Following the intersession, suggestions and interventions are provided to the clients. Consistent with the model's focus on client strengths, interventions are preceded with commendations that highlight client strengths and resources. The goal of therapy is that the client leaves the session with a self-defined positive outcome and reduced distress (Houger Limacher, 2003; McElheran & Harper-Jaques, 1994; Slive et al., 2008).

Current Service Description

Consistent with its roots, the EFC continues to deliver prompt, accessible and affordable counseling services to community members who walk in for self-defined mental health and behavioral issues. The services are offered at no charge. Hours of operation are 11:00am to 8:00pm Monday through Thursday, 11:00am to 7:00pm on Friday, and 11:00am to 3:00pm on Saturday. In order to continue to meet the needs of the changing community, the EFC provides a continuum of services designed to be the least intrusive possible. These services consist of a telephone crisis line, a mobile support team, a walk-in service, brief focused counseling, and facilitated access to the services of on-site partner organizations.

Walk-in Single-Session Therapy

The core service at the EFC continues to be walk-in single-session therapy. Clients arriving at the EFC complete a basic form that provides demographic information and outlines their reasons for accessing counseling. They are also provided with information about the counseling process (e.g., team approach, one-way viewing mirror) and the limits of confidentiality. Typically the wait time to see a therapist is less than twenty minutes. Counseling is delivered by a team of multidisciplinary therapists. One interviews the client while the other team members watch from behind the one-way mirror. When issues of risk and safety to self or others are present, therapists assist clients to develop safety plans, and in some cases make referrals to either the hospital or child protection services. Clients leave their sessions with specific practical ideas and plans that lead in the direction of problem resolution.

Focused Counseling

Another service offered at the EFC is the provision of on-site brief therapy whereby clients meet with the same therapist for up to five sessions on an appointment basis. Families that could benefit from brief therapy are identified both through the walk-in service and by other referral sources, including the city's mental health crisis services. The EFC provides assessment and treatment for children, youth and their families with situational, developmental or chronic and complex mental health concerns. The EFC provides approximately 300 sessions to 60 families annually. The frequency of session depends on the nature of the problems. Sessions may be closely grouped or spread out over time.

School Based and Outreach Counseling

Over the course of the EFC's 20 years of existence, the walk-in model has been extended to a variety of community settings where families could access services more quickly or where emerging problems were being recognized. In order to create a more responsive network of services connected to the Centre, assistance was initiated at two area elementary schools known to serve significant numbers of at-risk, high-needs families. School personel refer families who are typically struggling with poverty, family breakdown, and violence. Many families are recent immigrants to Canada. There are often underlying mental health concerns affecting the parents. As a result the children are also under a severe degree of stress. These children may develop behaviors that interfere with their ability to learn and that negatively affect their social interactions. The EFC annually provides service to 10% of children enrolled in these schools by offering brief counseling for children and their parents to assist families to resolve situations that are generating detrimental stresses. This intervention program aims to prevent problems from becoming more extreme and reduces the likelihood for more intensive intervention from child protection services, special education class time, and other more expensive interventions through the health system. The counseling assists parents to improve their parenting and coping skills. The program connects families with community resources geared towards stabilizing and improving their circumstances. Therapists teach children stress management skills while at school. Children improve their social skills and learn to interact positively with teachers and peers.

Time-limited provincial grant funding has also allowed for the provision of walk-in, group and focused counseling services in partnership with other community agencies. When funding is in place these services are offered at various agency sites throughout the city and give another option for families in the community who may have reduced access to transportation to the EFC. Through collaborative relationships and formal partnership agreements, the Centre has co-developed and facilitated a number of initiatives identified by the community to fill gaps in current services delivery options or areas of emerging community need. Examples of such initiatives include the provision of a therapeutic process group for women affected by domestic violence, a psycho-educational group for adolescents with challenging behaviors and their parents, and a school based experiential group for 6-10 year olds affected by various forms of trauma.

Community Resource Team

The Wood's Homes Community Resource Team offers telephone crisis and mobile response services that are connected to a broad network of other crisis mental health services. A 24/7 telephone support and crisis intervention service offers suggestions to alleviate immediate stress/crisis, coordinates with family members to plan for safety, and refers the families to appropriate community resources. Contact may be maintained with families until the crisis is resolved. Mobile crisis response visits are arranged on the basis of the nature of the telephone contact, the family's request and receptivity, or when the need for problem assessment via direct observation is indicated. The purpose of this mobile response is to provide rapid, accessible intervention at a key moment in order to promote safety for children, adolescents and families, to strengthen family coping skills and to enhance their capacity to function effectively in the community. These visits are provided as soon as possible and within 24 hours of telephone contact. They focus on family strengths and resources for reducing functional problems and diverting hospital contact and admissions.

Mental Health Collaboration

Psychiatrists have consulted at the EFC since its inception by participating as members of the walk-in teams. These psychiatrists, along with volunteer therapists who work within the city's health services authority, have added value to our existing services through their knowledge and connection to other formal mental health system structures and their familiarity with local programs, policies, procedures, and organizational culture. Their knowledge enhances the Centre's ability to support clients who require more intensive interventions or services as a result of high emerging risk to self or others, and also provide ideas for ongoing service development. As an example, clients presenting at a hospital emergency department with acute symptoms may be referred to the EFC rather than being admitted. Through collaboration with the city's health services authority, the EFC can assist with the diversion of these clients away from more intensive hospital-based services by providing increased access to preventive mental health services and reducing service fragmentation.

A vital clinical collaboration is the EFC's relationship with the health services authority's Mobile Response Team for adults at risk. When clients accessing the walk-in service are deemed to be at high risk due to a complex mental health concern, Centre staff can contact this mobile crisis team who will come to the Centre and meet with the client to determine next steps. This process allows for a further assessment of risk and smooth entry into the health services authority's mental health system if necessary. The Mobile Response Team also provides an alternative to inpatient services since they can follow up with the client in their home or the community as needed.

The EFC has also established other two-way pathways linking various mental health services. These include the local 24-hour crisis/distress phone line, the child protection emergency services phone line, and the hospital emergency room's psychiatric nurse on call. At-risk clients involved with these services are referred to the no-wait EFC walk-in service and, in turn, the walk-in service can refer clients to their services. While many of these clients benefit from a single-session of walk-in therapy to meet the immediate crisis need, those who require additional support can be referred to the appropriate services quickly and efficiently.

Another key relationship for the Centre is the ongoing collaboration with the mental health system's central intake and triage system. This intake and referral system helps to direct clients toward appropriate clinical services such as the EFC, and refers appropriate clients to the Centre's focused counseling service.

Teaching and Training

When the EFC began as a pilot program, everyone involved assumed an attitude of being a student of the processes required to develop a service innovation. Building a rigorous clinical model and being faithful to it across all types of clinical sessions allowed for reflection and a culture of continuous learning. This culture drew staff, volunteers, and psychotherapy students from various backgrounds to the Centre. Today the EFC is affiliated with a variety of local, provincial, and national teaching facilities and serves as a training venue for medical and mental-health disciplines including masters and doctoral students from applied psychology, nursing, clinical social work and counseling, as well as medical family practice residents. Regular in-service training is offered to volunteer community therapists and clinical supervision is provided for post-graduate professionals to meet licensing requirements for their professional designations. The Centre's clinical staff members offer training in the walk-in single-session model to interested and qualified mental health practitioners across the country.

What Success Looks Like

Client Satisfaction with the Service Provided

Of the approximately 2200 walk in sessions per year, 45% are provided to families with parent/adolescent conflict, 30% to couples with relationship conflicts, and 25% to clients who are seen individually, with the most common presenting problems being mental health concerns. Over time, the need to measure the effectiveness of the service became obvious, and the Centre experimented with various methods of determining success. The Session Rating Scale (SRS) (Duncan, Miller, Sparks, Claud, Reynolds, Brown, & Johnson, 2003) was eventually chosen as a performance indicator for single-session therapy. The SRS is a brief tool that measures the common factors predicting strong outcomes by highlighting the client/therapist relationship and reflects the trans-theoretical model utilized by the EFC. Keeping in mind that research by Asay and Lambert (1999), as well as Saunders, Howard and Orlinsky (1989), emphasized that the formation of a strong and effective alliance from the client's perspective was a good indicator of positive therapeutic change, it was determined that the SRS would effectively measure the strength of this indicator across the variety of presenting concerns, therapists and types of sessions that occur at the Centre. The SRS asks four questions that assess the client's level of satisfaction with feeling heard, understood and respected. A five-year analysis of SRS data collected from the walk-in service found average scores between 85% to 90% agreement with the four positive statements, indicating that a strong alliance typically developed in sessions.

Immediate Reduction of Level of Distress

The Eastside Family Centre's walk-in therapy service also asks clients to rate their level of distress before and after the session using a simple unmarked 10cm scale with 'None' at one end and 'Extreme' at the other (Duncan et al., 2003). The difference between pre- and post-session self-reported levels of distress is measured and used as another performance indicator of positive therapeutic outcome. Approximately 95% of all clients complete the Session Rating and Subjective Distress Scales immediately after each session. Annual analysis over the past five years indicates that clients report an average decrease in level of distress after their sessions of 20 - 25%. This decrease is considered statistically significant and implies that the session experience may be assisting clients to find methods to frame or structure their problems in ways that provide hope for change.

Another performance indicator is client perception of the responsiveness and accessibility of the Centre itself. Immediately following the session, clients are asked to evaluate their first impressions of the Centre by phone, rating their experience with the receptionist, with the atmosphere while waiting, and with the forms they were asked to complete on a five-point Likert scale. Clients' average ratings of their experience over the same 5 year period was between 4.3 and 4.5, suggesting relatively high levels of satisfaction related to the responsiveness and accessibility of the Centre itself.

Why Do Clients Return

In addition to the immediate feedback that clients provided about their experiences of the counseling sessions, the Centre became interested in why, on average, 30-35% of clients returned to the EFC each year. Some clients returned almost daily or weekly for a period of time, while others returned months or even years after their first single-session visit. As a result, Miller and Slive (2004), then Miller (2008) sought a more in-depth quantitative and qualitative response from clients about their experience at the Centre. Miller (2008) collected follow-up questionnaire data from 417 individuals who had received services through the EFC. The data indicated that 83.3% of the respondents were generally satisfied with the services they received. One quarter of respondents reported that the greatest strength of the Centre was the 'walk in' availability, while the second highest reported strength was having someone who listened.

Miller and Slive (2004) conducted telephone interviews with 43 clients 3 to 5 months following their walk-in session to determine if they were satisfied with the service and whether or not they felt there had been improvement in their presenting concern. They found that most respondents were satisfied or very satisfied with the service. In addition 67.5% of the respondents (29) reported some level of improvement and only three of the respondents (7%) indicated that things were worse. Again in 2005 Lawson, McElheran and Slive (2006) contacted 100 clients of the 37% who returned in a given year for one or more additional sessions. These clients reported that they connected with the service rather than with an individual therapist, they appreciated the therapy team approach and the advice they were given, they liked having a menu of suggestions, and they felt safe.

Finally, a customer satisfaction survey was completed in 2009 to solicit feedback from returning EFC clients to determine why they returned for services and their opinions of the services they received. Clients who attended and returned for an additional session between 2007 and 2008 were contacted by telephone. The first fifty (6% sample of clients who returned) to agree to participate were selected for the study. When asked what they most remembered about the services they received, 90% of the clients responded that they were pleased, satisfied or otherwise had a positive memory of their experience; 42% spoke of feeling heard, understood and supported; and 38% mentioned the level of professionalism and demeanor of staff.

Case Examples

The Harbor Family

Alex and Rhonda brought their children David, age 16 and Ellen, age 18, for a walk-in session at the EFC. The parents reported that David spent all of his time in the basement and on the computer, except to come up for meals. David was taking online education, as he did not want to be with other people. He stated that he preferred to be by himself and was not interested in close relationships, as he felt they did not last. He believed he would have to be in a public school for grade 12, but that was not until next year so he would deal with that when the time came. Alex was concerned that this was not good for David's well being and worried that David might be depressed. David had been taking an antidepressant prescribed by his doctor for many years. Rhonda agreed that she was worried about David, but she had other concerns, and was not sure how long she could handle remaining with the family. She explained that Alex recently "ran away from home" and they finally found him after a week at the local homeless shelter. She said the family talked Alex into returning home, but she feared he would run away again if he felt overwhelmed by stress. Rhonda also indicated that Alex had "run away" twice before during their twenty years of marriage.

Alex explained that some of the stress he experienced included being unemployed and not able to adequately support the family. He stated that he was a welder but had been unable to find work for the past nine months due to the recession. The family had gone through other periods of financial difficulty; they currently owed $8,000 in back rent and were facing an eviction notice. They also reported that they were on the verge of having their power and gas shut off and that they have experienced these stressors at other times as a family. Rhonda stated she worked at three jobs, but she did not have the qualifications to earn more than minimum wage. She said that she felt responsible for the maintenance of the family, and she could not do this anymore because each time Alex left it brought up issues of her own abandonment as a child.

Alex and Rhonda described Ellen as being very different from David. They saw her as very social and often expressing feelings of inadequacy, asking her parents for support to deal with seemingly simple tasks. She was four months pregnant and intended to have the baby, although whether she would keep the child or give it up for adoption was uncertain.

The family's physical presentation was disheveled. David's hair was not combed and he wore running shoes without socks. Ellen wore an oversized sweatshirt and undersized sweatpants while Rhonda wore a long "peasant" dress, no makeup and appeared very tired. Alex was dressed in jeans and a dark t-shirt. The family explained that they had been involved with many service agencies such as the family resource center in their community, and had received emergency financial support that helped pay for their damage deposit and a one-time rent payment. They described how they had applied to the local public housing authority but felt discouraged by the long wait to get housing. They did not feel that any service had been able to support them for a significant period of time; in turn they did not appear to meet the expectations or requirements set forth by those agencies for further support.

When the team met for the intersession break they wondered if coming to the EFC was another step in seeking help, with the strong possibility that the Centre would be part of a long line of services that the family had experienced as not being helpful. The team decided to focus on David's social struggles as the identified family problem. A typical intervention would have been to structure time for David to spend with other people, starting with regular family time. However, the team hypothesized that this would not contribute to change because David had been very clear that he was not interested in spending time with either his family or finding new friends. The therapist returned after the consultation break and commended the family members for their strength in remaining together for so long under such difficult circumstances. The various behaviors described by the family were reframed as their search for strategies to cope with many overwhelming challenges and that their behaviors made sense when looked at through this lens.

The therapist used a narrative orientation and externalized "Helplessness" as having been a pervasive member of the family for a long time. The therapist pointed out that David's isolation may have been a way to manage Helplessness, similar to Alex; running away, when Ellen frequently requested help, and when Rhonda considered separating. These behaviors were said to make good sense from the perspective that Helplessness had often led the family to the brink of chaos and break up. Each of these behaviors could be seen as a way to remain a family. The ongoing difficulty however was that the family remained on the brink of a disaster. It also left the family within a framework that was very depressing and hopeless. The team then challenged each family member to take a step against Helplessness and take a step instead towards standing up for themselves in support of the family.

The family seemed to accept this challenge. Alex agreed to clean the kitchen and the mess left by the pets so that the cooking area would be more sanitary. Rhonda said she would do the laundry that had been piling up for a long time so there was no more laundry on the floor. Ellen agreed to get her room ready in case they had to move, and to clean the living room and bathroom floors of animal droppings. David told the therapist and family members that he would clean the basement and a closet that was packed with stuff untouched since the family moved in three years ago. The therapist suggested that, as David cleaned, he should throw away some things that the family did not use or were broken.

The family's description of their living space (clothes all over and areas that had animal droppings) seemed to increase the grip of Helplessness that the family likely lived with on a daily basis. Therefore, their choices to stand up to Helplessness were acknowledged because these choices gave them the satisfaction of living in a cleaner more enjoyable environment.

Rhonda, who completed the session rating scale for the family, indicated that their level of distress had decreased significantly (from 9 to 5.5 on the ten centimeter scale) and that they felt respected and understood by the therapist. Five days later, Rhonda "walked in" to the EFC by herself to "check in" and make sure the family was on track. She said Alex was working, which was a major relief for the family, and that she had almost all of the laundry done. Rhonda stated that Ellen and David were making minor efforts to fulfill their agreements and that they were continuing to make progress. It appeared that Rhonda had greater hope for the future of the family.

Sarah

Sarah arrived at the EFC on a Saturday morning. She was visibly upset and stated that she had been awake all night. She wanted to talk about her 20-year-old son Jay who lived with her. Sarah was a single parent; her ex-husband had little contact with Jay. Sarah described how she had left her husband when Jay was four years old because of ongoing family violence. She went back to school, got a diploma in social work, and was working in a supervisory position in a local shelter for Aboriginal women. Sarah stated that she had grown up in a home that espoused Aboriginal values but that she no longer participated in many activities related to her culture of origin. On Friday morning she and Jay had had a serious disagreement about Jay's refusal to get out of bed and attend a class at the community college. Sarah believed that, since she was contributing to his school costs, Jay should follow her direction about school attendance. Jay told Sarah that he believed, because he was an adult, he did not need to tolerate his mother telling him how to run his life. The argument escalated and Jay hit his mother hard in the face. He left immediately and Sarah had not had any further contact with him.

Sarah answered the therapist's "why now" question stating that she could not bear to be at home alone without resolving the argument, that she was beside herself with worry about her son's future, and she was devastated that she was again a victim of violence in her own home. She felt terrible about her difficulties raising a son who could resort to violence so easily and who could not function on his own, and she stated that she was a "bad mother." When asked how she would know that it had been worth her while to come to the Centre, Sarah answered that, if the session were successful, she would be leaving with a concrete plan about how to find her son, get him to come home, and talk with him about how the fight had put a strain on their relationship. She explained that she was anxious to re-establish emotional connection with Jay but that she was frightened and concerned about her level of safety when another disagreement might arise.

The therapist for this walk-in session operated a highly successful private practice with a specialty in clinical hypnosis. He volunteered regularly at EFC in order to stay fresh with more generic counseling skills and to benefit from the ongoing learning opportunities that the team approach and regular in-service training afforded. After offering some reflections and commendations, and building engagement, he asked Sarah if she could sit back and picture having a conversation with an imaginary client at the shelter. He used some hypnotherapy techniques to assist her in relaxing and using her imagination. He then asked Sarah to "just chat" with her imaginary client, who had been struck in the face by a son. Sarah quickly engaged in the process and gave her "client" almost a dozen ideas about how to think about her situation and how to respond to it. The therapist took detailed notes, although he rarely did this in his other Eastside sessions. When it was time to take a break, he suggested that Sarah stay relaxed and not focus on anything in particular until he returned with comments from the clinical team. That Saturday morning was very busy and the therapist could not find another team member for consultation. He returned to Sarah and apologized for not being able to provide her with any other perspectives on her situation but offered to review his notes with her. She laughed and remarked that she was his "team" and that she had gained renewed faith in her ability to handle her upset and Jay's. As they reviewed the therapist's notes on the suggestions that Sarah had given her imaginary client, Sarah indicated which ones were a good fit for her, and she left with a solid plan. She reported a 5-point drop in her distress level and gave the therapist "full marks" (as she put it) on the Session Rating Scale.

Sue and John

Sue and John, working professionals with three small children, came to the EFC after Sue discovered John viewing pornography on the internet. Sue was at home on maternity leave after the birth of their third child, and while using the computer one afternoon she had been bombarded with pop-up advertisements for websites selling pictures and stories of what she saw as degrading sexual activity. When she examined the browser history she discovered that John had not only been visiting the sites but was also downloading pictures. She acknowledged that she knew of John's use of pornography when they met 12 years ago, but after they had married 10 years earlier he agreed to stop. Sue reported that she had caught him in possession of movies, magazines and internet pornography on different occasions during their marriage, and each time he had shown embarrassment and remorse, had apologized, and agreed that he would not use it again. Sue said that she felt betrayed by what she saw as John's blatant lying to her about pornography and wondered what else he was lying about. Sue's goal was for John to apologize and to demonstrate/prove to her that this time he is trustworthy. John appeared embarrassed and said he knew what he had done was wrong and that he was very sorry.

During the session both Sue and John talked about how committed they were to their family and to each other. Each was able to talk about their core values, common goals, dreams as a family, and each one's hopes for the future. Sue, however, wondered whether they would have a future together given John's continued betrayal of their vows by lying. She also said his viewing of other women in a sexual way made her question if she was not enough for him or if he was not attracted to her anymore. John was fairly quiet during much of the session, but he tried to reassure Sue that he was both committed and attracted to her and that he wanted to rebuild her trust. He seemed uncomfortable talking about this with a third party and apologized to his wife several times for his actions. John came up with the idea that he would quit his job out of town, stay home, give Sue all his passwords for their computer, or even forego the computer. Sue said that these actions might be a start, but these promises did not make her feel much better about their future given that similar promises had been made in the past. The therapist used systemic questions with the couple, exploring the way that they handled conflict and discovered some significant differences. Each was asked about their history and comfort level in addressing conflict in their relationship. Sue indicated that she grew up in a family that had clear, open and assertive conversation. She talked about boisterous conversations, disagreements and debates at the dinner table where she learned to speak up and to stand up to her siblings. Sue claimed that this style of conversation helped her to be a stronger person and to develop her career as an attorney. John described being raised on a farm in a more traditional family where there was significant emotional distance between his mother and father. He remembered that their dinner conversations involved focused listening but not questioning. When a topic was upsetting or a conflict arose between his parents, his father would go to the workshop. His mother would not pursue or continue the conversation, thus ending the interaction.

The therapist asked how difficult it was for John to speak up in the marriage or even in the session. John responded by saying how uncomfortable it was for him to talk about difficult topics, especially with Sue, whom he perceived to be more skilled in verbal communication. Thus, the pattern that had developed was for John to apologize and withdraw in order to end conflicts as quickly as possible. Sue perceived his withdrawal as a lack of commitment. This left her with feelings of sadness that she tended to express through anger and blame. During the session both Sue and John appeared to recognize that each time they had a serious conflict they never really resolved it. At this point the therapist took a break for team consultation.

When the therapist returned from the consultation, the couple had moved closer together and were holding hands. They announced that during the break they had continued the discussion and were feeling more hopeful about their future. During the intervention phase of the session the therapist praised the couple for their deep commitment to their marriage and their willingness to look at the broader issue of their patterns of conflict. Because they agreed to continue, after the session, to work at developing an alternate view of their conflict, the therapist commented that the team wondered how this might change the way they approach each other. The therapist offered a suggestion that the couple consider slowing down the change process by spending some time getting to know each other again through other aspects of their relationship, such as their friendship. The therapist stated that, by building some safety and trust, they might develop new ways of managing conflict. Following the therapist's comments, Sue and John said that they might find new ways to learn about and manage the other's communication styles, although both indicated they were not sure how they were going to find a unique style that worked for them. They said that the session was helpful and reported that their level of distress had decreased. They expressed a wish that the session had been longer. Sue and John walked in for two more sessions over the next six weeks and continued to work on building and strengthening their marriage. Each time they appeared closer to each other, more respectful of the other's voice, and described ways in which they felt closer to finding ways to manage the conflicts that arose in their marriage.

Where Are We Headed?

After 20 years the EFC has established itself as an essential component of a coordinated system of mental health service delivery. With the implementation of a cost/benefit philosophy in health and human services over the past ten years and the movement towards less intrusive community-based mental health services, there has been an increasing focus on service coordination, efficiency and accessibility. Through the use of walk-in single-session therapy for both acute and chronic mental health issues, the Centre has been able to provide therapeutic interventions, education, guidance, psychiatric consultation and referral to a wide variety of individuals, couples and families.

One way that the EFC has stayed relevant is to regularly go back to its roots; reevaluate the needs of the community and how to best meet them. One of the initial areas reviewed was whether the hours of operation (originally 1 to 9 pm) still met the needs of the clients who accessed the Centre. After reviewing 5 years of data, it became apparent that most clients were coming earlier in the day (75% before 5:00 pm) and that the hours of operation that were initially set to meet the needs of individuals and families after typical work and school hours might not be fitting as well as they once were. After some experimentation in the fall of 2009, on January 1, 2010 the Centre adjusted its hours to open two hours earlier in the day and to close one hour earlier in the evening. There was an immediate impact with an 11% increase in utilization from the previous year. This effort was also augmented by a marketing campaign designed to reach new Calgarians who might not know about the Eastside Family Centre, as well as community professionals who might refer clients. The EFC distributed over 20,000 brochures to local resource centers, schools, churches, libraries, hospitals, and community physicians. Additionally, the Centre ran advertisements in 12 quarterly community newsletters, two local newspapers, and a variety of local publications. The Centre also began to explore internet-based and social networking opportunities to connect a new generation of clients to the service, such as advertising on Facebook.

In order to meet the demands of a growing client base due to expanded hours and marketing, the use of volunteer therapists to staff the Centre had to be reconsidered. For 20 years, the EFC relied on mental health professional volunteers to support the daily operations of the walk-in service. However, over time there has been a gradual reduction in volunteer numbers as many of the original volunteers had begun to retire from the field and new professionals were not emerging in sufficient numbers to fill the gaps. The EFC reverted to a past strategy and advertised in the publications of the various professional organizations (social work, psychology, and marriage and family therapy) to recruit new volunteers for the centre. This advertising highlighted the opportunities for new professionals to receive supervised training and a variety of clinical experiences, and for retired professionals to remain connected to the field in ways that meshed with their reduced schedules and career changes. This strategy was rewarded as new social workers and psychologists saw value in the opportunity to accumulate the required hours for their professional licensing or to have ongoing and regular consultation concerning their professional practices. Similarly, a number of experienced and retired professionals are finding that volunteering at the EFC is an opportunity to remain connected to clinical work while providing guidance and support to new professionals.

Today's EFC leadership team members are participating in two community advisory committees for the development of community-based mental health services in the under-served northeast and southeast quadrants of Calgary. The experience and expertise generated at the EFC has positioned the Centre as a leader in community mental health. Its innovative ideas have informed the way mental health service systems are being developed and delivered.

This year the EFC thanked volunteers both past and present for their contribution to the success of the Centre, when it celebrated its 20-year anniversary. The Centre hosted a one-day workshop for therapists across the city that was facilitated by Dr. Arnie Slive, a co-founder of the EFC, which highlighted the single-session approach to therapy and the value of the walk-in model. The evening concluded with a celebration that honored the history of the EFC and looked forward to its continuing contribution the community.

Conclusion

For 20 years, the EFC has remained committed to the value of walk-in single-session therapy as an effective means of meeting the clinical needs of clients. However, over time it has become important to understand walk-in therapy in the context of the system of mental health services available to individuals, couples, and families. Many clients make use of a single-session of counseling and do not require further resources. For those who want (or need) more, the Centre has now become an effective treatment option for clients transitioning between levels of care, services, agencies, and systems to ensure that their mental health needs are met while they await services or need a "booster" session. The EFC has been able to positively impact gaps in treatment and challenges to effective service coordination by providing an immediate, accessible, affordable and effective community service designed to meet the identified needs of the clients they serve.

References

Amundson, J. (1996). Why pragmatics is probably enough for now. *Family Process,* 35, 473-486.

Asay, T, & Lambert, M. (1999). The empirical case for common factors in therapy: Quantitative Findings. In Hubble, Mark A (Ed); Duncan, Barry L (Ed); Miller, Scott D (Ed). (1999). *The heart and soul of change: What works in therapy.* Washington, DC: American Psychological Association (pp. 23-55).

Bloom, Bernard l. (2001). Focused single-session psychotherapy: A review of the clinical and research literature. *Brief Treatment and Crisis Intervention,* 1(1), 75-86.

Boscolo, L., Cecchin, G., Hoffman, L., and Penn, P. (1987). *Milan systemic family therapy.* New York: Basic Books

Duncan, B, Miller, S., Sparks, J., Claud, D., Reynolds, L, Brown, J., & Johnson, L. (2003). The Session rating scale: preliminary psychometric properties of a "working" alliance measure. *Journal of Brief Therapy,* 3(1), 3-12.

Duncan, B.L., & Miller, S.D. (2000). *The heroic client: Doing client-directed, outcome-informed therapy.* San Francisco: Jossey-Bass

Houger Limacher, Lori (2003). Commendations: The healing potential of one family systems nursing intervention. (Unpublished doctoral thesis). Calgary, Alberta, Canada: University of Calgary.

Hoyt, M.F. (Ed.). (1994). *Constructive therapies* 1. New York: Guilford Press.

Hoyt, M.F. (Ed.). (1996) *Constructive therapies* 2. New York: Guilford Press.

Hoyt, M.F. (Ed.). (1998). *The handbook of constructive therapies.* San Francisco: Jossey-Bass.

Hubble, M. A., Duncan, B. L., & Miller, S. D. (Eds.). (1999). *The heart and soul of change: What works in therapy.* Washington, DC: American Psychological Association.

Lawson, A., McElheran, N., & Slive, A. (2006). *Why clients return to a single session walk-in counselling service* (Unpublished manuscript). Woods's Homes Eastside Family Centre, Calgary, Alberta, Canada.

Lipchick, E. (2002) *Beyond technique in solution-focused therapy.* New York: Guilford.

McElheran, N., & Harper-Jacques, S (1994). Commendations: A resource intervention for clinical practice. *Clinical Nurse Specialist,* 8(1), 7-10.

Miller, J. K. (2008). Walk-in single session therapy: A study of client satisfaction. *Journal of Systemic Therapy,* 27, 78-94.

Miller, J., & Slive, A. (2004). Breaking down the barriers to clinical service delivery: Walk-in family therapy. *Journal of Marital and Family Therapy,* 30, 95-103.

Saunders, S., Howard, K., & Orlinsky, D. (1989). The Therapeutic Bond Scales: Psychometric characteristics and relationship to treatment effectiveness. *The Journal of Consulting and Clinical Psychology,* 1(4), 323-330.

Slive, A., MacLaurin, B., Oakander, M., and Amundson, J. (1995). Walk-in single sessions: A new paradigm in clinical service delivery. *Journal of Systemic Therapies,* 14(1), 3-11.

Slive, A., McElheran, N., and Lawson, A. (2008). How brief does it get? Walk-in single session therapy. *Journal of Systemic Therapies,* 27, 5-22.

Slive, A., McElheran, N., and Lawson, A. (2001). Family therapy in walk-in mental health clinics. In M. MacFarlane (Ed.), *Family therapy and mental health: Innovations in theory and practice* (pp 261-285). New York: Haworth.

Talmon, M. (1990). *Single-session therapy.* San Francisco: Jossey-Bass.

Tolan, P. H., & Dodge, K. A. (2005). Children's mental health a primary care and concern. *American Psychologist,* 60, 601-614.

Wampold, B. E. (2001). *The great psychotherapy debate: Models, methods and findings.* Mahwah N.J: Lawrence Erlbaum Associates, Publishers.

White, M., and Epston, D., (1990). *Narrative means to therapeutic ends.* New York: W. W. Norton.

Chapter 7

The Walk-in Clinic at the Community Counseling Service

Monte Bobele, Ph.D. and *Arnie Slive, Ph.D.*

The Community Counseling Service (CCS) originated as a practicum training site in the late 1970s at Our Lady of the Lake University (OLLU) in San Antonio, Texas. At that time, there was a modest master's training program in Community Counseling. The CCS, in reality, was a one night a week campus-based operation that provided limited counseling experience for graduate students in a setting that was used during the day by a speech and hearing clinic. It was fortunate that the speech disorders clinic had been constructed with treatment rooms that were adjacent to observation rooms with one-way mirrors. The mirrors and observation rooms made a live-supervision model possible. Clients were recruited from local churches, schools, and other informal sources. The CCS rarely served more than three or four clients a night. Students were limited to seeing a case or two each semester.

The OLLU master's program evolved in the late 1980s from its community counseling origins to a master's in Psychology with specialties in family therapy and counseling. Under the leadership of Glen Gardner and Tom Conran, the department developed a doctoral degree in Counseling Psychology, and the university accepted the first PsyD Counseling Psychology students in 1990. The doctoral program incorporated the training model developed at the CCS into its training at the doctoral level. The training model at the CCS was cited by one APA site visit team as the "jewel in the training crown" of OLLU's doctoral training program. With the increased enrollment that the move to professional psychology programs at the master's and doctoral levels required the CCS outgrew its shared location with the speech and hearing clinic. Eventually, the CCS grew to a six day a week operation that has, for the last 20 years, occupied a separate, community based facility about two miles from the main campus.

The CCS offers a sliding fee scale to make services available to the vast majority of our clients who have annual incomes below $20,000. The CCS shares a waiting room with a group of family physicians that serves the same low-income population. The CCS is open six days a week and assists clients either by appointment or on a walk-in basis. The creation of the walk-in service has increased the number of clients who come to CCS expecting a single-session consultation. Because our services have become well known in the community, many local agencies also refer lower income walk-in clients to us.

Most of the clients seen at the clinic are either self-referred or are referred by community agencies, friends, the court system, the University, or other schools. The clinic serves a largely Hispanic neighborhood with the majority of residents being Mexican-American. During 2009, CCS clients included 80% Hispanic, 12% Caucasian, 3% African-American, and the remaining 5% were identified as Asian-American, Native American, Middle Eastern, or "other racial/ethnic groups." A plurality of clients (44%) had an annual income of $5,000 or below, 14% were in the $5,100-10,000 range, 20% in the $10,100-$20,000 range, 11% in the $20,100-$30,000 range, 7% in the $31,000-$50,000, and the remaining 4% had annual incomes above $50,000. Although clients often call ahead to schedule an appointment or to inquire about our services, we rarely screen clients by complaint or diagnosis. This practice has worked well over the years. (We are indebted Teresa Correia, Anthony Nguyen and Bernadette Solórzano for compiling this data.)

Our students have benefited from exposure to a wide range of problems and clients. We routinely see a variety of ages, individuals, couples and families; we see LGBT clients; we see people with chronic mental health histories and serious chronic medical conditions contributing to other problems in living. In other words, our policy and practice is that we offer our services to anyone and everyone, whether they schedule an appointment ahead of time or walk-in for services.

At the time I arrived at OLLU, I (MB) had recently finished a postdoctoral fellowship at the Galveston Family Institute (Andersen, Goolishian, Pulliam, & Winderman, 1986). There I had become familiar with brief treatment models, live supervision, working with multiproblem cases, and other aspects of training that found a comfortable home when transplanted to San Antonio's Westside. Then in the early 1990s, I was part of an accrediting team that visited a family therapy training program in Calgary where Arnie Slive and others (Slive, MacLaurin, Oaklander, & Amundson, 1995) had established a walk-in clinic that served a multi-ethnic, multi-problem population. I was impressed with the model that had been implemented (Chapter 6). They assumed that each session could be treated as a self-contained episode and strove to provide maximum assistance at the time when clients were most in need of help. Their model permitted clients to be seen with no wait list and none of the usual intake hurdles.

After some discussion with colleagues in our psychology program, we decided to implement the walk-in procedure on a limited trial basis at the CCS in 1997. There were a number of factors that convinced us that such a model was a good fit with our clinic. Most importantly, we were fortunate that our psychology faculty embraced theories about psychotherapy that are derived from social constructionist premises. In a department that had more theoretical diversity, we might have been challenged to justify such a brief approach with our colleagues. The Psychology department's graduate programs and the CCS already had in place a number of resources that made a walk-in service possible. At the time we began offering walk-in services, three of us (Joan Biever, Glen Gardner and Monte Bobele) had extensive postdoctoral training in brief systemic forms of therapy. We had been teaching brief methods for several years. As we increased our faculty, one of the skills we looked for in applicants was either experience in providing brief therapies or a willingness to learn them. Additionally, we established a training/service delivery model that put supervisors and students in the CCS from 9AM until 9PM four days a week. These hours were important for a clinic operating a walk-in service.

Our clinic already routinely treated the first session as the beginning of therapy. In other words, we did not use the first visit as a screening visit or a diagnostic opportunity. We got right down to business. Our experience over the years was that about half of the clients who scheduled a first appointment failed to appear. We also found that half of the clients who did come for their initial visit and scheduled a second appointment did not return. Students were discouraged when their clients did not return. Faculty explained these "premature terminations" to themselves, and sometimes to students, as a result of novice therapists' difficulty in establishing a therapeutic relationship. We told ourselves that our particular population was unfamiliar with the nature of psychotherapy. We flirted with conventional ideas of resistance. We took refuge in data that the modal number of therapy sessions anywhere was one. We were occasionally comforted with these explanations.

At the same time, in light of the research about the frequency of short term planned or unplanned therapy, the fact that many clients came only once began to make sense to us. This body of research helped us begin to shift our thinking. It gave us a way to capitalize on our strengths in working from a brief model. It provided us with a way to talk to students about using momentary motivation. It gave us the opportunity to encourage students to focus on what could be gained in a single-session instead of attending to the failure of clients to return for therapy. It allowed us to hypothesize that it could be a sign of success when clients did not return after a first session. We were heartened by the results of a student's dissertation research that found that clients who did not return as expected had been satisfied with the help that they had received at the CCS (Scamardo, Bobele & Biever, 2004).

When we decided to pilot the walk-in model in the CCS, we limited it to the half-day that I was supervising a team of therapists. The prospective supervisees were informed that we were going to be trying something different with our cases. We notified our citywide referral sources about our new "single-session walk-in services" and the available times for walk-ins. Because we share a building with a group of family practice physicians with a common waiting room, we were able to post signs there announcing our walk-in service. Most callers to the CCS were informed about the walk-in services.

We found that the walk-in approach was a good and familiar fit with our clients. Many amenities offered to families in our neighborhood are available on an immediate walk-in basis. For example, the medical practice that we shared a waiting room with sees patients on a walk-in basis. Most of the Catholic churches in our neighborhood offer walk-in confessions. Many government offices such as the food stamp centers, child protective services, probation departments, and others allow clients to walk in for services. Barber shops, beauty shops, automobile garages, and many other institutions in our clients' lives operate on a walk-in basis. We believed that these contextual factors boded well for a walk-in counseling service.

Current Operation of the CCS

The CCS's large sign outside the building on a heavily traveled neighborhood street advertises, in both Spanish and English, that services are available on a walk-in basis. The CCS has not abandoned an appointment-based system at this time; it currently operates a hybrid system. When prospective clients call ahead to inquire about the clinic's services, our staff gathers basic information about the caller, schedules an appointment, and informs them of the walk-in hours. All clients, whether they phone ahead or walk in, are given the option of a walk-in session or a session by appointment. Prospective clients who request appointments are scheduled at available times with one of the treatment teams. Prospective clients are also routinely informed of the possibility of simply walking in without an appointment.

We have struggled with a number of ways to eliminate the downtime no-shows create, given that only about half the new cases scheduled actually show up for their first appointment. We have found that the arrival of a walk-in case helps to fill down-time. All teams are on call to handle walk-in cases. Clients who arrive at the clinic without an appointment rarely have to wait more than an hour to be seen. Such a long wait is rare but comparable to the wait at walk-in public health clinics or emergency rooms.

When clients enter our clinic, they complete the standard forms providing demographic and billing information. Before the session, clients meet briefly with a graduate assistant who explains how we work (e.g., this is a training facility; we use a team approach; we use a co-therapy model; sessions are routinely video recorded) and sets the fee. Additionally, they complete a form that asks a number of questions to orient the therapists and the client on immediate concerns and problem solving: "What is the problem that we can help you with today?" or "What are your assets?" We negotiate problem definitions with clients from a single-session perspective. For example, low self-esteem, depression, poor communication skills, or DSM-IV diagnoses are not useful problem definitions for us. We work with clients toward problem definitions that are behavioral, observable, specific, and under the client's control (Walter & Peller, 1992). Typically, therapists inform the clients at the beginning of the session that many clients decide that one session is sufficient but that later in the session they will be given the option to walk in again or make an appointment for another session. If they chose to schedule a subsequent appointment, they may see the same two therapists or the same team.

Training goals

The CCS serves as the primary training site for our master's and doctoral Psychology students. Our graduate programs require that students complete approximately 16 hours of practicum training each week in the CCS during the first year and a half of their degree programs. At any one time there are approximately twenty-five students providing therapy every week. The numbers of students working in the CCS have proved to be sufficient to provide appointment-based therapy as well as the additional walk-in services.

We employ a team approach with six therapists and a supervisor on a treatment team. The team's structure follows the procedure outlined by the Milan team (Selvini-Palazolli, Boscolo, Cechin, & Prata, 1978). Typically, the supervisor and most of the team members participate in the session from an observation room connected by closed circuit television, while two team members interview the client. The supervisor and observing team members are able to make suggestions by telephone during the course of the session. More typically, toward the end of the session, the entire team meets together to compare observations and plan the closing of the session.

The walk-in service at the CCS provides our graduate students with training in extremely brief, walk-in therapy that is not available anywhere else in the Central Texas area. Students develop skills that enable them to offer these services in a variety of settings after they complete their graduate training. The collaborative nature of our training and treatment provides opportunities for students to see the immediate effects of their efforts.

Training programs that emphasize long-term approaches to therapy may be doing their students an unintentional disservice by not providing them with an opportunity to see the outcomes of their cases. For example, during a team discussion preparing for clients scheduled for later in the day, we reviewed the outcomes of the previous week's sessions. Two of the three cases that this team of therapists had seen for initial sessions the previous week were sufficiently helped in those session that they said so, and told the therapists that they did not think they would need to come back. The third case had decided at the end of the session, which was her third, that she had a handle on her situation, and would not need to come back any time soon. One of the students, a third semester master's student, said, "This doesn't happen on any of my other teams. We hardly ever see cases that have ended successfully." She went on to explain that in her previous training experiences, the sessions emphasized rapport building. Lengthy conversation that was not necessarily directed toward client goals was not discouraged. The student contrasted this with her current team approach in which each session had a clear focus and worked toward goals mutually defined by client and therapist.

We have been surprised to find that the influence of the single-session work has spread to other clinical settings where our students receive training. Students find that they have learned the skills to provide timely assistance to clients in these other clinical contexts. An early example of this was a case that a student worked with on another CCS team that was not oriented to walk-in/single-session work (Bobele, Lopez, Scamardo, & Solórzano, 2008). Selia had been working with me on the walk-in team for several months at the time she was referred a Spanish speaking case on another team. The Latina client was concerned about whether her own history of childhood sexual abuse would inevitably lead to abuse of her own children. A few hours after the session, which had been focused on identifying strengths and resources, the client called Selia with a report of first steps she was already taking to insure a healthy, loving relationship with her sons. Chapter 4 of this book presents a number of examples of our students' walk-in single-session work at other local agencies such as the local sexual abuse crisis center and a large government mental health facility that demonstrate the application of these ideas in other settings.

Ways that the CCS is incorporated into the Psychology training program Practicum

The CCS is the first clinical training experience for all graduate Psychology students at OLLU. For master's students, the CCS provides an intensive, supportive training experience for the first two semesters of practicum. Members of a team may be master's students or doctoral students. Our training model encourages heterogeneity of experiences in each practicum team. We have found that beginning students learn more quickly if they work with more advanced students who can model collaborative learning. More advanced students benefit from the challenges of helping beginners learn the ropes.

Nearly half of OLLU's graduate students are Hispanic and this diversity is reflected on the CCS treatment teams. The OLLU Psychology department has developed a nationally recognized program that trains bilingual/bicultural psychologists. As one aspect of that training program, we offer one or two half-days a week of therapy in Spanish. This service also benefits from the walk-in service offered by the CCS. Having a large number of Spanish speaking therapists also makes it likely that teams that provide services in English will have bilingual therapists who can serve Spanish speaking clients when they walk-in.

Pre-Practicum Class

Master's students take a practicum preparation class at the end of their second semester in the program. This class follows classes in general counseling theories as well as two courses in systemic therapies. The pre-practicum class is oriented toward providing students with the necessary skills to begin clinical work in the CCS specifically, and other settings in general. The systemic therapy and pre-practicum classes emphasize strength-based, brief approaches to helping clients resolve problems. In the pre-practicum class, students are asked to observe several teams in the CCS and write a paper describing their impressions.

Assignments in other classes

The CCS is also used as a practicum placement for undergraduate Psychology students. Undergraduates sit in on team meetings and behind the mirror on ongoing cases. Undergraduates are invited to participate actively in team discussions and frequently become quite sophisticated in formulating cases. Undergraduate Psychology students who do a practicum in the CCS often go on to graduate programs at our university or others.

The capstone master's systemic therapy course in our department makes significant use of the CCS. Students are required to develop an analysis based on a case they treated in the CCS. This case analysis is presented at the end of the semester to the rest of the class. The cases selected for presentation are, more often than not, based on single-session cases that came to the clinic on a walk-in basis.

Research

The CCS is an established site for our doctoral students to gernerate their disseration research. We have had several dissertations and professional presentations based on clinical work with walk-in/single-session therapy from the CCS.

Example from CCS: Shawne's and Brandy's Case

The following case illustrates the use of single-session, walk-in principles at the CCS. These principles, as described in Chapter 3, are the following:

1. The session is only one hour.
2. Within that hour, we have a whole therapeutic session.
3. We narrow the database to the immediate problem.
4. We look for common factors.
5. The therapist's therapeutic influences are tempered with pragmatism.
6. The session involves a consultation with other therapists.
7. The therapists focus on what the client wants from the session.
8. We seek to understand the client's resources.
9. We explore the client's previous attempts at a solution.
10. We make use of the client's own motivations.
11. We commend the client.

Marcos was interviewed by two therapists on a team supervised by Arnie Slive. The team behind the mirror was comprised of a mix of doctoral and master's students at various levels of experience. The team observed the case in a room adjacent to the therapy room over a closed circuit TV. One of the co-therapists, Shawne, was a Latina doctoral student. Brandy, her cotherapist, was a Caucasion master's student in her first semester of practicum training. This was one of her very first sessions.

Marcos was a 20-year-old Mexican-American who lived near the clinic. Marcos originally walked into the clinic one morning accompanied by his mother and girl friend. There were no therapists available at the time, so they were invited to return to the clinic to be seen a couple of hours later. When they returned, Marcos' mother and girlfriend waited in the parking lot for him. Marcos and his girlfriend (whom he occasionally referred to as his wife) had a two-year-old daughter. At the time of the interview, Marcos was living with his mother. His girlfriend and daughter lived with her mother. He had been attending trade school, but had to withdraw because of excessive tardiness. He had recently lost two jobs because he lacked reliable transportation, but was trying to do landscaping to earn a living. During the interview, Marcos reported a history of self-inflicted cutting, but had not engaged in this behavior since becoming a father.

Steps In Developing A Single-session Context

Rapport

We are mindful that research on the common factors indicates that the client-therapist relationship accounts for nearly a third of the change in successful therapy (Hubble, Duncan, & Miller, 1999). We view the establishment of a necessary and sufficient relationship as essential to begin moving the client in a therapeutic direction. We are also open to the ideas that such a relationship can be established in a relatively short period of time, and that the establishment of a therapeutic relationship is a dynamic, evolving process that takes place over the entire course of the therapeutic encounter. In many cases, clients come to their first session already highly motivated to begin the process of change and may require only minimal relationship building to proceed with therapy. In this case, Marcos had begun establishing a therapeutic relationship with the CCS earlier in the day when he and his family had dropped in to inquire about services. We have found it useful to think of the therapeutic relationship as being much broader than the client's relationship with the therapists in the consultation room. We think of the therapeutic relationship as extending to the staff answering phones, the receptionist, and the team of therapists working with the client. Research at the Eastside Clinic in Calgary found that clients cite their relationship with the facility, not individual therapists, as the reason for return visits after weeks or months of a previous session. Our antidotal evidence supports this premise, too.

The transcript of the session that follows has been edited to fit within the space confines of this chapter. Some of the dialogue has been edited to improve readability.

Problem Definition and Negotiation

Marcos came to the CCS with a potentially overwhelming number of problems. Pay attention to the patience demonstrated by the therapists. Therapsts working within a walk-in/single-session model do not speed through a session. Nor do they need to try to move Marcos faster than he is willing or able to go.

After a brief introduction to the clinic and its procedures, Marcos summed up his situation.

Marcos: Uh, I'm looking for some answers. I've been having a lot of problems with jobs and stuff. I had two jobs, and they both fired me.

Shawne: Oh, what were your jobs?

Marcos: Uh, the one in the morning was landscaping all day. And, the one at night was night plumbing. So if people would have problems at night, you go everywhere in San Antonio. Like people would have a problem in the middle of the night with their plumbing. Because it does happen, and it happens often, more than people think.

Shawne: Yeah.

Marcos: It's just a big ol' mess in the middle of the night. I was a plumber's helper, and since I didn't have a car, he doesn't want me.

Shawne: Oh, ok.

Marcos: Basically I'm in a hole, and I can't, I just can't do anything.

Marcos went on describing a perfect storm of unfortunate events that had happened in the last few weeks. During this recitation, Marcos kept his head lowered, his eyes on the carpet just in front of his feet. It would not have been unreasonable for the therapists and the team to have interpreted this body language as evidence of a severely depressed mood. Just before the client left this session, however, he explained his lack of eye contact to the therapists.

His brother-in-law was also his business partner in his lawn care business. His brother-in-law borrowed his car and wrecked it beyond repair. Marcos depended on the car to get to his jobs. His brother-in-law stole money from him. His brother-in-law had a drinking problem and was unreliable, frequently not showing up to help Marcos with their landscaping jobs. As Marcos became more comfortable with the therapists, he added that at an earlier point in his life, he had been a "cutter," and had been hospitalized. Then, he disclosed to us that his best friend had been murdered the previous month, on Marcos' birthday.

Marcos: And like, I tried to get my friend to help me cut yards to get a business going.

Shawne: Uh, hmm.

Marcos: Uh, I gave him half the money, and he split with the other half and I got to fix the yard by myself. And it's just one house, but it's like an acre yard that the person has. I just feel like the world has screwed me over, and I yelled earlier. I told, I told my wife and my mom to just leave me alone, and I came here. I listened to them, and I'd rather not go off. 'Cause I used to be a cutter, and I used to cut myself. So, I'd rather not do that anymore.

Shawne: Oh.

Marcos: Since my daughter was born, I'd rather help myself instead of, like when we were younger. She's [his girlfriend] been with me when I was like 14, and I cut myself. That wasn't really great. I went to the hospital and they stitched me up so that was it.

Shawne: That's one of the things that I guess your mom and your girlfriend were worried about, too. That you might do something like that. And, you said you hadn't done it in a long time. So how did you, how have you managed to stop doing that?

Here Shawne is highlighting successful coping strategies that Marcos uses to avoid cutting again.

Marcos: Because I don't want my daughter to see my scars.

Shawne: Oh.

Marcos: 'Cause if she cuts herself, then it's like really sad.

So, Marcos' devotion to his daughter is important to him, and helps him avoid repeating problems he had in the past.

Marcos: Today has just been a bad day for me. My friend got killed on my birthday actually.

Shawne: Oh my goodness.

Marcos: Like, he was one of my friends that I made money with. Yeah, I did everything with him. I can't find a partner that I can make money with me, like he did. Yeah, and they shot him in the back.

Brandy: That must have been really hard.

Marcos: Yeah, my friend was a good guy. He didn't deserve to get shot. And, it was over his daughter. He may have been slow, he may have been, you know, a little on the off side but he was the coolest person I knew.

Marcos has presented the therapists with several problems: he lost two jobs, his brother-in-law wrecked his car, his best friend was recently murdered, he had a psychiatric history that included cutting. He had also been attending a trade school but was expelled because of excessive absences. He had not been able to go to school without a car. Marcos went on to liken his situation to a Biblical character.

Marcos: And like, I don't how to say it, when I got out of high school, I didn't have no money. I didn't have a car. I didn't have nothing, and somehow I made it. And, then I lost everything. It's like, have you ever read the Bible? Like that dude, Job? God took everything away, and he still praised

God. Right now, that's how I feel, like that guy, Job. I hope God gives me my stuff back.

Asset Inventory

An important feature of single-session work is creating, with the clients, an inventory of their strengths and resources that can be recruited to help them get back on track. Marcos has offered several examples of his coping skills. Following a phoned-in suggestion from the team, Shawne continues this process with Marcos.

Shawne: That's the rest of the team watching, and sometimes they have questions, or things that they are curious about, and they'll call in. And, one thing they're curious about is, with all these things that you say you've got going on, how have you managed to do as well as you're doing?

Marcos: Not giving up!

Shawne: Not giving up?

Marcos: Like, I think, 'cause my uncle put it to me like, "you got a will, there's a way." I don't stop trying, but earlier I was breaking down and crying. And they [his mother and girlfriend] took me here. And, I still feel like crap, you know.

Shawne: Yeah.

Marcos: But, like, I haven't broke down like that since I was really little. They're really worried about me, and that's why they took me here.

Shawne: But, it sounds like you do keep trying even when these things happen to you. That, like you said, you lose everything and then you overcome it, and you keep on. And you work, and it sounds like you take care of your daughter, and you take care of your mom.

Marcos: But that's the reason I'm working—because of her. If it was just my girlfriend, I would be like, "Oh well, she gives me more problems than I need," you know. I'd rather have my baby there. My baby makes me happy more than anything. I'll smile at her even though I'm probably dying, and she was right there.

Shawne: Yeah. That's a lot of stuff. That's why I'm still like wondering how, with all that stuff, you're still even able to get up, and come back over here? I mean you could have said, "yeah, I'll be back," and then . . .

Brandy: Not show up.

Shawne: But, you still came back. That, to me, shows that you're the kind of person that doesn't quit, and a responsible guy. I mean, if you say you're going to do something, then you're going to do it.

Marcos: Yeah, I just didn't want to act stupid in front of my daughter. 'Cause CPS [Child Protective Services] is, they're really sensitive about having a whacked out dad. And, I just don't want to be one of those whacked out dads. They have to have counseling, or something …'Cause I would actually go crazy if they took my daughter away. 'Cause that is the only thing that makes me keep on going.

Brandy: After all the things that are going on with you, the thing that's still in your mind, that I see, is your daughter. And, that's the only thing you're still worrying about. You're not even worrying about yourself, it seems like. You want to change things for your daughter. (He nods yes).

The therapists did an excellent job of taking stock of the assets and strengths that this client had in order to help Marcos' to move toward a resolution to his problem. We believe this case highlights how clients are always changing. It is remarkable that Marcos used resources available to him, as we see below, during their two-hour wait for the session. After Marcos and his family left the CCS earlier in the day, his mother took him to see the priest that he had grown up with.

Marcos: I talked to my [priest], after I left here, 'cause they [his mother and girlfriend] thought ya'll were going to give me counseling right away when we came here earlier. And, like that's what they thought. And when we left, she took me to St. Jude's and I talked to, I talked to a priest.

Shawne: Oh, ok.

Marcos: And he was like, like this dude used to talk to me when I was in diapers. He was like, "It's alright, Marcos." I haven't seen him, in like, 11 years. He said "You grew up!" and I was like, all I could say was, "I don't have a car" (laughs). That's all I could say, and I don't have nothing to show for it right now.

Shawne: And, so did he say anything to you that was particularly helpful?

Marcos: Yeah, "Pray and God will help you." And, "If you've given up, then you've let the devil win."

In order to begin setting the stage for problem resolution, the therapists elicited more examples of strengths and assets already in play in Marcos' life. He described his responsible work ethic and his responsibility toward his daughter and his family.

Marcos: But I hold two jobs so I can pay my mom and my girlfriend. 'Cause I got to buy diapers, I got to buy wet wipes. I got to buy lots of stuff for her—even her clothes.

Shawne: Yeah.

Marcos: She's growing, and my mom needs food for the house and other stuff like that. And, then I lost my second job—it wasn't today—it was the day before.

Problem Resolution

Marcos went on to describe his dilemma and the reason for his current distress. His girlfriend's brother, who was also his employee, was becoming increasingly unreliable. The brother had wrecked his car leading to the loss of the two jobs for want of transportation. He had also been coming to work late and drunk. Marcos had been considering firing him, but was sensitive to how his girlfriend might react.

Marcos: How are you gonna' know like he's a drinker? I'm the boss. How are you going to call me in the morning and tell me "I didn't know that I was going to have that much to drink." And, I was like, "Are you serious? Are you coming to work? Are you just going to stay there? Are you gonna…? —You're fired dude. That's it!"

Shawne: Uh hmm.

Marcos: He said, "How can you do this? I call you. . . I'm your brother." I said, "How are you going to do this to me? Not come to work?" I just don't know what to do. If I fire him, he has two kids, I have one. If I fire him, she's [Marcos' girlfriend] going to get mad at me. I just, I don't know what to do. I would like ya'll's opinion. Should I fire him? I don't know. That's one of, that's one of my problems.

Then, Marcos provides the therapists with language that will help them help him resolve his dilemma.

Marcos: I don't know what to say about this. I think I should [fire him] because that would be a good boss's decision. But, that would be a bad brother-in-law decision. You know what I mean? Like it's like a split down the middle, like I don't know what to do.

Shawne: Uh hmm.

Marcos: So, I didn't go work today. I actually came here. This is where they took me. My girlfriend told my mom, which I obey my mom's every word. I just came here. I just don't know what to do from here, now.

Shawne: Yeah. Well it sounds to me like you have an idea of what you should do.

Marcos: A little one but like . . .

Shawne: I'm sure you've heard this before. They say you shouldn't do business with family. I mean we've all done it, don't get me wrong. I mean we've all done it, and we think "Man, how to we get out of this now? Without making so-and-so mad, and hurting this person?" And, it can be hard. So I can understand why you having such a hard time with it. But, like you said, you also have a child to take care of and raise, and, that you want to make money for. And, it sounds like you make pretty good decisions when it comes to those things. And, knowing that, that you're a good decision maker, and you're a responsible person, I think you are the best judge of what to do in that situation. And, I think the reason you're having such a hard time is 'cause you already got the decision made. And, you know what might be the consequence, or the result of that decision.

Marcos: I'm not going to argue with him, if I make my decision.

At this point, the therapists have framed his dilemma as one that realistically balances his obligations as a boss with those of a brother-in-law. The team phones in a suggestion that calls upon Marcos' respect for his murdered friend's advice.

Shawne: That was the team, and they had a couple of questions. They were curious because you were looking for feedback and for advice. They were just wondering, if you could ask the friend who passed away for advice, what do you think he would tell you about what you're going through now?

Marcos: Man, I miss that dude. He would tell me to ignore it, and keep on going. And then we'd kick it and play basketball or something. That's what he would tell me. I guess I know what ya'll are talking about because that fool was a really close friend of mine.

Shawne: It sounds like it; the way you talked about him. Even though you talked about him just for a moment, we could tell that that he was important and still is to a certain degree in your life.

At this point the therapists told Marcos they were going to take a break to consult with the team. During the consultation break, the team outlined strengths that they saw in Marcos, and some suggestions about how Shawne and Brandy might encourage Marcos to hold his head high, in spite of the seeming plague of problems that had visited him recently. Marcos had said several times in the course of the inteview that he had come to the CCS for feedback. One of the principles of walk-in/single-session therapy is to find out what the client wants, and give it to him. So, the therapists framed their remarks, when they returned, as feedback.

Shawne: Well, it took a little bit longer, but the team really had a lot of feedback and a lot of things they wanted us to say to you. First and foremost, they understand that this has been a bad day for you. You've got so many things going on. You're talking about possibly firing your brother-in-law, the money issue, and then the loss of your friend. It seems like you've had a lot of losses.

So even though you may not agree with what the team's feedback is, we did want to share it with you. They feel that, in spite of all that stuff, you have a lot going for you. They have a lot that they want to praise you for: you're responsible, you put your daughter first, even though you've got all these things going on for yourself. That you worry about how other people are going to feel even though you need to do what's right for you as well. You're looking at your brother-in-law, and even though you said he's been a bad employee, you're still concerned about him and his family. And so, they were really impressed with everything you're managing to do in spite of the losses. And they recognize that because it's been such a bad day you might not see it that way right now, but . . .

Marcos: Yeah, I understand.

Shawne: They wanted us to share that with you because they were so impressed. They felt that you have a lot of things to really hold your head up high about. You're able to still put your daughter first, and take care of her, and worry about all those things that a father does. Even though you say you can't be there, you say you're still working to provide her diapers, and food, and clothes, and all those things that are important to raise a healthy baby. So, it sounds like you have an idea of what you should be as a father. You're doing those things by working and providing. By trying to do the best, even with the situation as it is. So they were very impressed with how you really want to set that good example for your daughter. And, so they wanted to share that with you.

Marcos: Yeah, that's nice

Shawne: And, to let you know that you do have a lot of things to hold your head up high about. And, they also thought that the reference you made to Job really did fit with your situation. His story was a story of perseverance. Things got really, really bad, and he felt that the weight of the world was on him. Yet, he persevered, and the struggle was hard, but in the end he came out on the...

Marcos: Top.

Shawne: Yeah, came out on top. So, they were like, "Wow, that really does sound like what Marcos is going through today."

As the hour was drawing to a close, the team phoned in with one more suggestion to help Marcos come to a decision.

Shawne: *(Phone buzzes).* One thing the team had mentioned earlier, and what I want to share with you before we wrap up for today is. . . When you talked about your brother-in-law, it sounded like you had already made a decision. So, maybe the best thing for you to do at this point is to figure out the best way to talk to him that's going to make you feel okay with it. You know what I'm saying? Do it in a way that you think, you know with respect. And, he'll have to deal with his feelings but . . .

Marcos: Yeah that's true.

Shawne: You want to say it in a way where you feel, "I did it the right way, I did it in the best way," and that's all you can do.

Marcos: Yeah, just 'cause he didn't work out right, I don't have to feel bad.

At this point, it appeared that Marcos had talked out his dilemma with his family, his priest, his therapists, and even his deceased best friend. The consensus that he heard was that he was a a responsible person with obligations to his family. He recognized that firing his brother-in-law was going to be difficult, but it was a responsible "boss's decision."

Client's assessment of the session

A critical aspect of walk-in/single-session work is determining whether the client received the help that they sought. The question of future sessions was left up to Marcos.

We are careful not to imply that clients need more help than a single-session can provide. Nor do we think that clients need to come back on a weekly basis. We believe that we communicate hope and optimism when we let clients make a determination about whether or how soon they would like to return. Our experience has also suggested to us that when we offer future appointments, sometimes clients agree, but then don't show because they are already feeling better. We sometimes think clients agree to future appointments to please us, not because they think they need one.

Shawne: And now that you're a little bit calmer, and you've thought about it, you can do it in a way that is more professional, like an employer would do.

Marcos: Yeah.

Shawne: 'Cause you've got to take care of yourself.

Marcos: Yeah, I'm letting you know something—don't hire him. Thank you for talking to me.

Brandy: You're more than welcome to come back either as a walk-in client, or make an appointment, if you like. I don't know if you found this helpful, but you can set up another appointment. It's completely up to you.

Marcos: Yeah, I'll probably do that. [Take advantage of the walk-in service.] I probably should have said this in the beginning. It's like an everyday thing with me. I've got a problem, a problem with women. I feel comfortable talking with guys.

Shawne: So if you came back, you'd like a male counselor?

Marcos: Well, with ya'll . . . I was pretty mad, and I let it all out, so I guess it didn't matter. That's why I couldn't look up. I'm sorry. I guess I could go ahead and set up another appointment with ya'll.

So Marcos' lack of eye contact was not a symptom of depression, but a shyness around women. Had he been given a choice, he probably would have said he preferred talking to male therapists. The team was surprised that he wanted to make another appointment before he left. We also hypothesized that when he agreed to schedule a follow up appointment, he may have been trying to reassure the therapists that they had been helpful, and he did not want to insult them. We thought that the session had been sufficient, and Marcos had met his goals for the consultation. He called several days later to report that he was doing better and would not need to come in after all. He was reminded about the availability of the walk-in service if he should need it.

Summary

This chapter has provided a description of how a walk-in single session service has been implemented in a university training clinic. The CCS differs from some of the training contexts that are present in university environments. The CCS is not the official counseling service for university students. However, in addition to its service to the community, the CCS offers counseling free to OLLU students, faculty, and students. The availability of such a training opportunity has benefited several constituencies in San Antonio. The citizens of the Westside of San Antonio have an excellent, easily accessible clinic that provides a variety of mental health services in a timely manner, frequently with no appointment necessary. Graduate Psychology students have an opportunity to receive live supervision while working with a variety of multiproblem clients in a real life context. Faculty and students have an excellent resource to develop new clinical approaches and conduct research. A number of doctoral dissertations have come out of research conducted at the CCS.

The CCS has taken advantage of its unique geographical and cultural context by explicitly encouraging the use of brief approaches to therapy and creating a means by which clients can walk in and get immediate assistance. In spite of the fact that the CCS continues to operate largely on an appointment basis for new cases, the ongoing training in treating each case as having the potential for being a single-session has influenced much of the clinical work done there. For example, the CCS offers therapy and supervision in Spanish four to eight hours per week. The "Spanish team" always has a few team members who have been trained on other teams to work from a walk-in single-session position. Prospective Spanish speaking clients are informed about the availability of walk-in services may arrive without an appointment for a consultation with the Spanish team.

Chapter 4 presents several clinical examples of our student's work in applying walk-in/single-session therapy in the CCS and in other settings across the city.

References

Anderson, H., Goolishian, H., Pulliam, G., & Winderman, L. (1986). The Galveston Family Institute: Some personal and historical perspectives. In D. E. Efron (Ed.), *Journeys: Expansion of the strategic-systemic therapies* (pp. 97 -122). New York: Brunner/Mazel.

Bobele, M., Lopez, S. S.-G., Scamardo, M., & Solórzano, B. (2008). Single-session/walk-in therapy with Mexican-American clients. *Journal of Systemic Therapies,* 27, 75-89.

Hubble, M. A., Duncan, B. L., & Miller, S. D. (Eds.). (1999). *The heart & soul of change: What works in therapy.* Washington, DC: American Psychological Association.

Scamardo, M., Bobele, M., & Biever, J. L.. (2004). A New Perspective on Client Dropouts. *Journal of Systemic Therapies,* 23, 27-38.

Selvini-Palazoli, M., Boscolo, L., Cecchin, G., & Prata, G. (1978). *Paradox and counterparadox.* New York: Aronson.

Slive, A., MacLaurin, B., Oaklander, M., & Amundson, J. (1995). Walk-in single-sessions: A new paradigm in clinical service delivery. *Journal of Systemic Therapies,* 14, 3-11.

Walter, J. L., & Peller, J. E. (1992). *Becoming solution-focused in brief therapy.* New York: Brunner/Mazel.

Chapter 8

Narrative Practices at a Walk-in Therapy Clinic

Karen Young, MSW

The Walk-in Clinic

For over eight years, Reach Out Centre for Kids (ROCK) in Ontario, Canada has opened the doors of our three walk-in clinic sites that serve three communities within our region. Each site has one eight-hour day a week designated to walk-in services thereby offering an opportunity for immediate access to a single-session of therapy at times when people are most in need. The clinics also serve as the "front door" to the agency so they function as the access point for any of the other services, such as ongoing therapy, treatment groups, or psychology services. The clinics are well advertised to the community through brochures at key referral sources such as doctors offices, schools, and on the agency's website. Before initiating the walk-in clinics, the agency had a more traditional method of intake that involved prospective clients calling an intake coordinator, completing a telephone interview and then being placed on appropriate waiting lists. Many people were waiting up to two years for further services. Although the agency does still have waiting lists for services that are beyond the walk-in clinic's scope, such as family therapy, groups, and psychology services, the wait for therapy has been reduced to a range, depending on the time of year, from 4 to 6 months.

The clinics are available to any families with children between zero and eighteen years of age who live within the agency's catchment area. There are no fees for service at the clinic, although clients are encouraged to make a one-time donation. In research (Bhanot & Young, 2009) we asked, *Who are our clients?* The findings suggested that clients with a wide range of mental health-related concerns (e.g., anxiety, anger problems, relationship problems, and depression) access ROCK's walk-in clinics. On average, clients had endured these problems for a year before they accessed services at the clinic. Our research also explored the question *Why do they come to our walk-in clinic?* Clients' responses suggested that the most popular reason for coming to ROCK's walk-in clinic was the recommendation of others (e.g. school, doctor, friends, etc.). The second most popular reason for coming was quick access to therapy. Finally, the third most popular reason was to access further services (e.g., individual counselling, family therapy, etc.).

In each walk-in site there are three to five therapists and counsellors, plus a supervisor, working each week. When clients arrive at our clinics, they are asked to complete an information letter and a questionnaire. The questionnaires were designed to reflect important brief therapy concepts (Young, Dick, Herring, Lee, 2008). These pre-session questionnaires set the stage for conversations that strive to elucidate the problem and to find hope, new ideas and knowledge about how to proceed. They help to recognize their abilities, skills and accomplishments, and use these in relation to the current problem they are experiencing (Epston, 2003; Young, 2006). After the questionnaires are completed the receptionist brings the clients to an available therapist who then sees the person/family for a session that usually lasts about one and one half hour. Therapists work alone, with co-therapist, or sometimes, with an outsider witness group (White, 2000). During the session the therapist openly takes notes on a Summary Report form that is photocopied and given to the family at the end of the session. Clients are given an evaluation form and asked to complete it at the end of the session (for all forms see Young, et al, 2008).

Information from Evaluations and Statistics

The number of families seen at the agency's walk-in clinics in the year 2008 to 2009 was 1500. This number has grown since 2001 when it was approximately 1000 families. Generally, 50% of clients are referred for further servies. Therefore about one-half of the families come to the clinics and receive a single session, which they experience as enough at the time. The percentage of clients who come more than once to the clinic is 27%.

About 50% of the clients who attend the clinic return completed evaluations after the session. What we have learned from these evaluations is as follows. The walk-in experience was reported to be a very positive resource for families. The majority of clients, averaging 89%, felt the session assisted them with dealing with the problem. Most clients, about 90%, felt that, before leaving the clinic, they had developed a plan to address the problem and were committed to carrying out a plan. A small percentage of respondents said that the service was disappointing in some way. This generally was in regard to wait times for further services. Approximately 92% of respondents said that they would come back to ROCK if the need came up in the future.

We have conducted surveys of other service providers in our community in order to obtain feedback about the impact of the walk-in clinic on their services and clients. We have received very positive feedback that indicates these providers appreciate the immediacy of the clinic, the quick access to therapy for their clients, and the opportunity for service with our clinic staff.

Research

Research was undertaken over 2008 to 2009 in order to evaluate the effectiveness of ROCK's walk-in clinic (Bhanot & Young, 2009). Although our walk-in clinic had provided brief therapeutic intervention for thousands of clients, and anecdotal evidence suggested that these interventions have been quite successful, an empirical outcomes-based evaluation of the walk-in clinic had not been conducted.

The purpose of the research was two-fold. The primary purpose was to conduct an outcomes-based program evaluation of ROCK's walk-in clinic. In particular, the effectiveness of the walk-in clinic was assessed by determining the extent to which walk-in sessions were producing the desired goals/outcomes. In addition, we wanted to gain a better understanding of the types of clients who came to the walk-in clinic, their reasons for coming, and what clients learned during the sessions.

The study was conducted using a pre-test, post-test and 2-month post-test design. The participants were 408 clients who accessed ROCK's walk-in clinics between October 2008 and April 2009. A pre-test questionnaire was added to the pre-session questionnaire already being completed by clients. Questionnaires were designed for both parents and children. Clients, after completing both questionnaires, proceeded to their walk-in session. Upon completion of their session, the therapist asked the clients to complete a post-test questionnaire. If clients consented to being part of a two-month follow-up, an investigator contacted them via e-mail or phone two months later.

The results suggest that a walk-in session produces a number of desired outcomes for clients. In particular, the results of the paired-samples t-test indicated that after their session, clients were significantly: 1) less worried, 2) feeling more competent about their skills as parents, 3) more confident in their ability to resolve/manage the problem, 4) more knowledgeable about available resources, and 5) had more ideas about how to resolve/manage their mental health problem.

Clients were also asked what they had learned during the session. When clients' responses to this open-ended question were analyzed, eight different themes emerged: 1) increased self-awareness, 2) awareness of the impact of the problem, 3) increased awareness of resources, 4) more general knowledge about the nature of the problem, 5) more knowledge of general strategies to help deal with the problem, 6) knowledge of specific techniques to manage mental health issues, 7) better communication skills, and 8) parental knowledge that children were willing to get help.

At the two-month follow-up, 100 clients responded. There were 26 clients who reported the original presenting problem was completely resolved. For the 74 clients for whom the problem was still a concern, they were still: 1) significantly less worried, 2) more knowledgeable about resources, and 3) had more ideas about how to resolve and/or manage the problem. Clients' responses suggest that they used fewer negative coping strategies and more positive coping strategies at the post-test. Since 26 clients reported that the problem was no longer a concern for them at the two month follow-up, the post test questions were modified somewhat to increase their applicability. In this case clients were asked to specify the extent to which the walk-in session helped to reduce or increase various outcomes. The findings suggest that the walk-in session had a significant and positive impact on a number of outcomes.

Walk-in Philosophy

The therapists who work at the walk-in clinics represent many diverse backgrounds, training experiences, and preferences for how to create therapeutic conversations. As therapists, we are informed by narrative therapy, Solution-Focused therapy, cognitive behavioral therapy, and a range of other ideas and practices. However, we have discovered that we all share many foundational philosophical ideas about people, problems, and how to be useful to those who come to consult with us. The following points are a short list of some of these beliefs and assumptions:

- People know when they need help.
- It's best to offer therapy when people are ready and asking for it rather

than when wait lists allow for it.

- Many people can benefit from a single-session and may not need more sessions.
- Many people will use sporadic single-sessions when they want help.
- Many people will also need a referral for ongoing services at the agency.
- Everyone is multifaceted, with many versions of problem and solution events.
- When people come for therapy they are unable to resolve a current problem/dilemma because they are limited by their current knowledge and understandings of their situation.
- People have knowledge, abilities and skills that can be discovered and developed in ways that can assist them to resolve current struggles.

We strive to be respectful of people's preferences and values. We are interested in joining with people around their agenda and concerns in ways that step away from the usual conversations they have been having about the situation and create a unique conversation that can bring forward new possibilities. We think it is important to find opportunities to assist people to question what they routinely think and do (White, 2007). We ask questions that create the possibility for discovering new ideas, knowledge, and skills. Our focus is on affirming people's strengths, on finding their resilience, generating hope, and facilitating learning.

We like to begin the meeting by saying something like: "We are ready to work hard with you for the next hour or so to help with the concerns that brought you here. Many people find that they benefit from one session here. If you do need more therapy we can provide that" (Rosenbaum, Hoyt, & Talmon, 1990). These words create optimism and hope that this conversation can make a difference.

The Beginnings of Brief-Narrative Therapy

Between 1995 and 2000, after seven years of study, training and practice of narrative therapy, I began to develop ways of practicing narrative therapy in situations where there was only very brief contact with clients. I began to notice the various practices that were most useful in quickly creating conversations that lead to the development of what we might call strength stories, or subordinate storyline development (White, 2007). I had the opportunity to develop these ways of practicing further when I began working at the walk-in therapy clinic at ROCK in 2001. Over the past 9 years I have discovered many ways of using narrative practices at the clinic (Young, 2008; 2006).

Narrative Philosophy and Approach at Walk-in Clinics

I have found that the presence of narrative thinking and practices greatly reduces the potential risk for rushed, and therefore less meaningful, conversations at our walk-in clinic. Narrative practice lends itself to "brief but deep" conversations. By deep I do not mean in depth assessment and information gathering. I mean conversations that are deeply meaningful, and therefore create and sustain new ideas, conclusions, visions, and hopes. We never know if the people we consult with will ever come again, so we must commit to making the most of each conversation.

The assumptions that guide my narrative practice at the walk-in clinic include the following ideas. Experience is subject to interpretation and meaning making that has many influences. It is multi-storied, with dominant and subordinate stories or narratives. Identity is fluid not fixed. It is relational, changes over time and between contexts, is influenced by internal narration, and has historical, present, and future possible meanings. Problems exist outside of people, between relationships and within contexts. The person is not the problem, the problem is the problem. People engage in actions or initiatives that reflect conscious purpose and intentions guided by their values, beliefs, commitments, preferences, hopes and dreams. People have knowledge, skills, talents and ability to take initiatives to reduce or resolve problems. And finally, people struggle with dilemmas and problems because they are limited by the "known and familiar," their usual ways of thinking and acting, but there are other ways of thinking and being available within the what is "possible to know" (Vygotsky,1978; White, 2007).

These guiding assumptions shape my actions within my therapeutic conversations with clients in the following ways. I am listening and curious—in a "not knowing the answer to the questions" (Freedman & Combs, 1996) position. I am being transparent and collaborative, like a learning partner. I am having conversations that externalize or unpack problems, separating the person's identity from the problem (White & Epston, 1990). I am curious about what people value and prefer for their lives, and what their skills and abilities are. I find their subordinate storylines and develop their details (White, 2007). My questions are aimed at story expansion, developing thick descriptions and richer meaning, guided by a "thin/thick metaphor" (Geertz, 1973).

The terms thin versus thick description are borrowed from cultural anthropologist Clifford Geertz (1973, pp. 6-7, 25-28). A "thick description is one that is inscribed with…meanings" and finds linkages between "the stories of people's lives and their cherished values, beliefs, purposes, desires, commitments, and so on" (White, 1997, p.15-16). I am asking questions that assist people to move from their known and familiar to what is possible to know, by facilitating learning through incremental questions (White, 2007). I document people's thought by doing my best to take down their exact words, often reading the words back to them during the conversation (White & Epston, 1990).

The questions that arise from the type of curiosity, guided by these assumptions, are aimed at the development of thick descriptions and rich meanings. These descriptions are generated through interviewing in ways that listen for what I call what is "in-the-shadows," or what Michael White terms "doubly listening" (White, 2004, p. 53). Discovering and making meaningful the subordinate or alternative stories in people's lives creates a new place for the person to stand, a platform from which they can see new possibilities in relation to the problem that brought them to the walk-in clinic (White, 2004). These conversations fall outside of the usual ways of thinking and speaking and, therefore, open up new possibilities. It is within these "unusual conversational territories" (Young, 2006, p.3) that I attempt to navigate. These are not technique driven, fast paced conversations. Instead, they appear slower. This may seem counter-intuitive in the context of a single-session, but my experience has been one of slowing down to speed up. The high volume of people attending the clinic could invite conversations that do not spend enough time on any one theme to develop its meaning. However, I want to linger long enough in important themes and moments to create meaningful conversations.

Re-membering Conversations

One of the most powerful ways to develop or *thicken* meaning in a conversation is to engage in *re-membering* conversations (Young, 2008; Young, 2006). In my conversations at the walk-in clinic, I often make use of White's re-membering practices (White, 2007 &1997; Hedtke & Winslade, 2004; Russell & Carey, 2002). Shortly, I will offer examples, through edited transcripts of sessions, of ways that I have used these ideas and practices in a single-session of therapy.

If we think of our lives as having "members," we can then think of people who have featured significantly in our lives, have been a source of inspiration to us, and have stood with us as members of our lives (Myerhoff, 1982). The purpose of re-membering conversations is to link what people value—important beliefs, principles and commitments—to those persons who have contributed significantly to the development of these values.

To explore what it is that a person values—the principles, beliefs, and commitments that guide their actions—I might use questions such as: "What do you think this action might express about what you care most about?" Or, "When you say that you are 'not a quitter' what values, beliefs, and commitments are reflected in this?" I ask about how these values show up in the person's life—other ways of being or actions that reflect these beliefs. I find out about the history of these values. How did this person come to embrace these beliefs? Did they see them expressed by someone else? Is this person from the past, present? Is he living or deceased, or fictional or famous? Who was that person? I may ask a question such as: "Can you tell me a story that would really describe how these values showed up in that person's life?" Then I might ask: "Can you tell me how this inspired by you in your own life and actions?" And, "What do you suppose it would be like for this person to know that they contributed to your life in this way?" "What might they say if they were here now?" "What might it be like for them to witness the expression of these values in your life now?"

Re-membering practices "provide the opportunity for persons to experience their lives more richly described through the identification and exploration of the history of their preferred knowledges and skills of living" (White, 1997, p. 59). I achieve this goal by carefully listening for "identity conclusions" (socially constructed conclusions about our own and others identities, White, 2007, p. 107) that people most often express through categories of personal strengths, characteristics, and qualities, and then "unpacking" these conclusions with particular care to link them to those persons who have contributed significantly to the development of these identity conclusions. This takes what is a thin description of a characteristic to a thicker description of it. If we think of life as a *membership*, we can consider these conversations as a way to "re-*member*" these people into the client's life (White, 1997). The initial characteristic is not replaced, but is expanded. What is achieved is "story expansion" not a story "replacement" or a "re-framing," which are completely different practices. These explorations answer the question: "Who stands with you, and in what ways?"

I believe the impact of these practices reduces the sense of isolation that often results from the problems people experience. When used at the walk-in clinic, these conversations can create an immediate sense of being less alone. Problems often separate people from their sense of themselves—being the person they prefer to be, the one who is living in ways that are guided by cherished values and commitments. In a single-session, re-membering practices can powerfully re-connect people with this sense of themselves. It provides them with inspiration about how to respond to the problem and how to proceed forward with their lives. My understandings of these possible effects from re-membering conversations are confirmed by one Bob's participation in a research project. His comments will be shared after the following transcript.

Stories

I saw Bob for a single-session while providing training at another agency that provides walk-in services to adults. The first part of the session included a conversation about "The Depression" that Bob had been struggling with for many years, "Its" effects on his life, and some of the ways in which he had attempted to reduce the influence of "The Depression" on his life (White, 2007). In the excerpt of the conversation that follows, Bob says that he is not a quitter. I became interested in developing this concept in relation to the values and principles this statement, "not a quitter" stands on. I was also interested in understanding what the history behind this may be, particularly as it relates to re-membering his life. I hoped that a re-membering conversation would put Bob more in touch with who stands with him in this struggle and would more richly describe this value and the member's contributions to it, thereby making his presence more available to him.

Bob: But, well, I'm not a quitter…quitting is a major no-no, it's not an option…. that's what's in me.

Karen: What do you think that relates to in terms of things you believe in, values, or principles that you have that relate to not quitting?

Bob: I don't know. I really don't know.

Karen: What kind of commitments do you think you have to yourself or to others in your life that keeps you going on this road to not quitting?

Bob: I really don't know. Quitting is just not a viable option. It's not a conscious thought…(pauses) but if it was a conscious thought it would have to be about a lot of the things I believed in growing up and people that I admired then, that it wasn't that quitting was not an option.

He begins to move from not knowing to knowing.

Karen: Could you say some more about that? People that you admired and things that happened when you were growing up…like going back in time and finding those things in the past that relate to this not quitting?

Bob: There's people that I know in the marital arts, and in competition, they just keep on going even if you made a mistake, because if you don't, you lose respect.

Karen: Like respect of the other people, or of yourself?

Bob: Respect from the judges and others there . . . the person is seen as - well, at least they tried . . . and they get points for keeping going, and they are admired for this.

Karen: Are you a person who has admired that, have you admired people who keep going?

Bob: Absolutely. I've done some work with some people who I really admire and who aren't quitters.

Karen: Who are they Bob?

Bob: Well the first person I remember is a person I worked with, John....

(Bob told a story of this man who had really contributed a lot to fairness and speaking up in the work place, who taught him about being even-handed. John respected Bob for his creativeness and his trying hard...taking initiative.) Then I ask:

Karen: I just wondered if he were here to comment, what he might say about this journey, this struggle with depression, and about keeping going, not quitting. What do you think John would say about that?

(I'm inviting Bob into a re-membering of John into his life.)

Bob: He'd say: "Keep on trying."

Karen: What would he say about how you've done things so far do you think?

Bob: I think he would be very supportive. But another thing, a person who has been really good for me is my teacher from China who has taught me Tai Chi.

(Another rich story comes forward. Bob tells about his teacher's many accomplishments and how he recently read an article that Bob wrote for a journal which was about people being heroes without even knowing it, about people standing on the sidelines, cheering, and how they really help, and are actually heroes...and he related all this to his struggle with depression and his teacher really liked the article and told him so.)

Bob: And that really means a lot, I believe its one of the things that has kept me going, and not quitting. There is nothing wrong with there being problems, but you need to just keep on going....

Karen: It sounds like he has been an inspiration to you and that this has helped you to sustain the not quitting.

Bob: Absolutely. Things like that really help me to appreciate what I've been able to accomplish . . . that really helps.

Karen: So Bob, have you felt John and your teacher standing with you on this journey?

Bob: Yeah, very much so. I've felt their supportiveness. It's been encouraging....

Karen: What do you think your teacher would say about your journey and all its challenges?

Bob: He'd say: "Keep on plugging…each day is a battle, keep on trying, each day is a mental battle…."

One and a half years later, in research conducted on single-sessions of therapy (Young & Cooper, 2008), Bob provided the following comments to the researcher about this session: "And she asked…have you known people like that? And the answer obviously is 'yes', but now she's the first one that's really come out and asked that question . . . like (who) would be standing beside me… encouraging, to continue to not quit . . . I hadn't even thought about that before that time, but it applies . . . Well in my mind, before that, I hadn't really thought about what they would think. I mean it was nice for me to know . . . and, you know, I've thought about it a number of times since." So not only was this meaningful for Bob in the moment, clearly it had lasting impact. I understand Bob's comments to reflect a reduced sense of isolation and a re connection with important values and commitments in his life. This was meaningful and made a difference.

Re-membering practices can be of great assistance in conversations with people who have lost people in their lives whom they loved and cherished (Hedtke & Winslade, 2004; White, 1997; 1988). I can engage in conversation with someone experiencing loss and sadness about a loved one who has died and vividly and powerfully reconnect their lives through re-membering questions.

Jay, age 14, and his father Ken came to the walk-in therapy clinic on the suggestion of Jay's school counsellor, who was concerned about his grief over his mother's death. Jay's mother had taken her own life about two years before. Ken was in the meeting for the first few minutes and then left as Jay expressed a preference to talk on his own. In setting the agenda I had learned that Ken wanted us to talk about "how Jay blames himself for it (mother's death), which isn't true. But that's what he feels sometimes." Jay agreed, saying that he wanted to "Just kind of to talk about my mum, and that part about feeling responsibility, to talk a bit about that."

Karen: I can only imagine how tough that must have been….(pause) Can you tell me something about what some of the effects have been on you of this?

Jay: I don't know... (pause) Well, well the world's not as bright as it used to be.

Karen: The world's not as bright. Does your mom being in your world brighten up your world more?

Jay: Yeah.

Karen: Would it be okay if we talked a bit about her? Like you introducing me to her?

Jay: Yeah.

Karen: What was she like? Can you tell me a bit about how she brightened up your world?

Jay: She's an amazing woman. She always knew what to say and she always knew how to comfort me. She was always there.

Karen: What kinds of things would she say to you? You said she really knew what to say?

Jay: She always had a story for everything. Every time I had a problem with something, she had a story to go with it, an experience she had, and like how she had dealt with it.

Karen: When you think of all the stories that your mum told you, is there one that stands out the most?

Jay: Probably the biggest one was ….

He tells a story his mom told him. Then I ask:

Karen: When people tell us stories, there's often a word or a sentence or something that really hangs around for us the most from a story. Is there a word or two from those stories? Or a feeling?

Jay: A feeling.

Karen: If you were going to describe that feeling . . . is that like a soothing feeling or a comforting feeling or a….

Jay: Calming . . . A calming feeling.

Karen: I was wondering, from all of what you learned from her, from the kind of way that she was. Do you think some of the way she was kind of rubbed off on you?

Jay: It rubbed off on me, I guess.

Karen: How did it rub off on you?

Jay: I don't know. My friends . . . I'd be that one . . . you know, let's not do this...that's not a good idea . . . Helping . . . And listening to them. . . .

Karen: So you learned this from mum? *(Jay nods)* Do you think she knew that you were caring with your friends and wanting to help them and be a good listener?

Jay: Yeah.

Karen: If your mom was in the room with us right now, what would it have been like for her if she'd heard you say those things...like helping people and being caring and a good listener and that you learned those things from her? What do you think that would be like for her to hear that?

Jay: I don't know…. *(pause).* I think she'd be happy.

Karen: Do you know why she'd be happy to know that?
Jay: That her son learned to be a good person.
Karen: I'm going to write that down . . . "That her son learned to be a good person from her."
Jay: Yeah.
Karen: Learning to be a good person.... So she'd be happy to know that you'd learned this from her. Would it be kind of like her leaving a legacy, with her son, of being a good person in the world? That she would know that that she wasn't here for nothing—that she left behind a son who she taught all about how to be a good person too?
Jay: Yeah. I think so, yeah.
Karen: Have you ever thought about that before?
Jay: Not really.
Karen: What's it like to think about that now? To think that you might be living out some values that your mum had about how to be a good person in the world.
Jay: It makes me happy.

Jay tears up. There is a pause in conversation, then...

Karen: I wonder if we might try to make some guesses about if your mom was sitting here now and I say, "Diane, this has been a really hard time for Jay. He's been really missing you and the brightness you brought to his life. Is there a story or some words you would want to share with him?
Jay: "Don't give up".
Karen: "Don't give up." What would she say don't give up on. Don't give up on what?
Jay: I don't know, just, I guess *(Pause)* Don't give up on myself.
Karen: She'd say don't give up on yourself. If I was to ask her, "Well when you say don't give up on yourself, what would you see him doing that would say he's not giving up on himself? How would you know?" How would your mom know that you weren't giving up on yourself?
Jay: That I was doing the best I could. Being the person I should be.
Karen: What would she see that would tell her you're being the person you should be?
Jay: I guess, that I'm still helping. Trying to help people.
Karen: So when your mom sees you doing that, she'd know "okay he's keeping going." What do you think.... if your mum were here, and she heard your dad say that he understands you feel some responsibility for what happened. What do you think her words might be about that? What position would she have on you seeing yourself responsible in any way for

what happened? Do you think she'd be for that, or completely against that?

Jay: No. She'd be completely against it!

Karen: She'd be completely against it. *(Nodding).* What do you think she would guess it would be like for you if she knew you were taking responsibility for that?

Jay: She would know how hard that would be. Too much grief.

Karen: Too much grief for you . . . . Would she think it was fair or unfair, just or unjust, or something?

Jay: Unfair.

Karen: She'd think it was unfair . . . . Do you think she'd have some understanding of how it happened? How this idea got going that it was somehow your fault. Do you think she'd understand it?

Jay: *(Nodding)* Yeah. *(Crying)*

Karen: What do you think she'd understand about it?

Jay: Why I blame myself. I got angry with her and I never got a chance to apologize. Just, not being able to tell her I'm sorry.... It's my biggest regret...

Jay is crying. There is a pause.

Karen: Is it okay if I ask you another question or two Jay?

Jay: Okay.

Karen: So, I'm thinking about what you told me about how your mum really knew you, she *got* you. Right? *(Jay nods.)* I wonder if she was here and I said to her, "Diane, Jay was showing some anger to you. You saw that and you know him so well. Looking at him through your loving eyes, as a mom, did you know that he felt sorry? Even though he didn't say it, he didn't have a chance to *yet*, did you already know?".... What do you think she'd say?

Jay: She could read me like a book.

Karen: So when she was reading you like a book, what was she seeing about you being sorry?

Jay: She *knew* I could never stay angry at her. Every time we got into a fight I would always come back and apologize to her.

Karen: So, she would have known that you were coming to apologize at any time. Is that right?

Jay: *(Crying, nodding).* Yeah.

Karen: Yeah. She knew. I bet you she could even imagine what the apology would sound like in her mind. How did you usually apologize to her?

Jay: I go up and hug her and say I'm sorry.

Karen: What would she say?
Jay: "It's okay".
Karen: She'd say "It's okay Jay."

Pause in conversation.

Karen: So Jay, if she were here, seeing how much regret about not having a chance to say the "I'm sorry" to her. What do you think she'd say about this now? If she were here, do you think she would try and lift this responsibility from your shoulders?
Jay: Yeah.
Karen: What words do you think she might used to do that?
Jay: I think like, "It's ok, I already knew you were sorry."
Karen: Yeah.

There is another pause. We have been talking for over and hour.

Karen: Could I summarize some things we've talked about today? *(Jay nods.)* You told me at the beginning that the world was brighter when your mom was in it because of how amazing she was, and how understanding of you she was, and how she calmed you with good advice and good stories. You said that you learned things from her about how to be caring and a good listener and helping other people. And you said that she'd be really happy to know that you learned those things from her. You said that if she were here she would say "don't give up on yourself, be the person you should be" and that she would know you'd be doing that because you'd been still helping others. Is this right? *(Jay nods.)* Yeah. And, you said that she would be completely against the idea that you were in anyway responsible for her death because she would know how hard it would be to think that, and she'd say that it's too much grief Jay. You told me that she could read you like a book and that she knew that you could never stay angry at her, that you would always apologize, because that's what you always did. And that when you did apologize, like always, that she would say "It's okay, Jay." And you said that if she was here today listening to this conversation that she would say, "It's okay, I already knew you were sorry." She'd try to lift the sense of responsibility from your shoulders. Do you think she'd do her best to do that? *(Jay nods.)* I do too, from everything you've told me about your mom.
Karen: What was it like to talk about these things today Jay? To talk about the things I just summarized back to you. How was that for you?
Jay: It was a lot. It was a lot of stuff . . . Sad . . . Happy . . . but good.

Karen: Do you know what the good part about talking about these things was?
Jay: It's just really good to talk like this....

After this session I wrote up the summary that I offered Jay in the session and mailed it to him in a letter. I believe that sending summaries of conversations to people will potentially assist them to stay connected to the new understandings and ideas generated in the session (White, 2007, White & Epston, 1990). I often write letters to people who have attended the walk-in therapy clinic for this reason. I then saw Jay and his father, Ken, three weeks later at the walk-in clinic. I had suggested that they come back to check in concerning how Jay was doing. The following letter is a summary letter that I sent to them after that session. As it summarizes our conversation, it will provide a clear sense of the session's content.

> Dear Jay and Ken:
>
> I was glad to have had this opportunity to meet with you both today and witness the ways you have found to change your relationship to one that is closer and more connected. You both said that this closer connection helped you each get through these last 2 years.
>
> I was also pleased to have the chance to read over and talk in person with you about the summary letter I sent you of the last session because I think it sparked some interesting conversation today.
>
> Ken you agreed that "for sure" Jay learned about being a caring person from his mom. You told *many* stories about the ways now and in the past that Jay has demonstrated his caring to others. You said that Diane would often tell you about comments and stories from others that she heard about Jay's kind acts, and that she would tell these stories to you, all the while smiling, and clearly so proud of Jay and the personal values and commitments he lives by. She knew, you told us, that this had to do with the kind of mom she was to Jay—that she had contributed to this.
>
> Jay, you told today about the importance of your connection with your grade 8 teacher and how much you have learned from him about being a giving and inspiring teacher. He has hugely contributed to your future picture of being a teacher with the values he has, which are like ones you have already. He is someone you talk to, who shares wise words and stories.
>
> Jay, I found out from you today that a way that you keep going, that you get up on some of the hard days, is by making sure that you see and notice the small acts of kindness that actually do go on in the world around you each day, and to be a part of this. That it keeps you going forward in your life to be engaged in your own acts of kindness to others.

Like those ways you have learned from your mom and from your teacher.

I feel lucky to have met you both. Come back any time if you need or like to. I learned from you both about how people can get through hard things, together, and by keeping true to what is most important to them. Thank you.

Sincerely,

Karen

I did not have any further contact with Jay or Ken after this second conversation. They both expressed feeling confident that Jay was doing alright, that he was moving forward in his life in ways that he, his dad, and his mom are proud of. I told them that they could come back to the clinic anytime if they wanted to. They strongly indicated that this process had been very useful and that they would not hesitant to come back if needed.

Summary

The walk-in therapy clinic at ROCK is providing unique and much needed services to the community. Parents, children and youth are making use of the clinic primarily to access a single-session of therapy when they most need it. Our agency's evaluation research has begun to demonstrate positive client outcomes. The agency will be continuing with further research on our clinic's effects and outcomes. I believe that narrative practices bring the potential for deeply meaningful and useful conversations to the context of a walk-in therapy clinic. These practices are a good fit with brief, single-session, walk-in clinic work. In particular, the narrative practice of re-membering conversations has assisted me to have conversations with people who are struggling with problems, such as ongoing depression and grief. These conversations reduce isolation and re-connect people with what has been temporarily lost—their sense of themselves and their stories of rich, sustaining, contributions made to their lives by others and to another's life by them. This provides them with inspiration about how to respond to problems and how to move forward with their lives in ways they prefer.

References

Bhanot, S. & Young, K. (2009). *An evaluation of Reach Out Centre for Kids walk-in clinic.* Unpublished manuscript.

Epston, D. (2003). Notes from *Inner-viewing of Narrative Interviewing,* Workshop at the Hincks-Dellcrest Institute, Toronto, December 8-9.

Freedman, J. & Combs, G. (1996). *Narrative therapy: The social construction of preferred realities.* New York: W.W. Norton & Company.

Geertz, C. (1973). *The interpretation of cultures.* New York: Basic Books.

Hedtke, L. & Winslade, J. (2004). *Re-membering lives: Conversations with the dying and the bereaved.* Amityville, New York: Baywood Publishing Company, Inc.

Myerhoff, B. (1982) Life history among the elderly: Performance, visibility and remembering In J. Ruby (Ed.), *A crack in the mirror: Reflexive perspectives in anthropology.* Philadelphia: University of Pennsylvania Press.

Rosenbaum, R., Hoyt, M.F., & Talmon, M. (1990). The challenge of single-session therapies: Creating pivotal moments. In R. A. Wells & V. J. Giannetti, (eds.). *Handbook of the brief psychotherapies* (pp. 165-189). New York: Plenum Press.

Russell, S. & Carey,M. (2002). Re-membering: Responding to commonly asked questions. *The International Journal of Narrative Therapy and Community Work, 3,* 23-31.

Vygotsky, L. S. (1978). *Mind in society: The development of higher psychological processes* (M. Cole, V. John-Steiner, S. Scribner, & E. Souberman, Eds.). Cambridge, MA: Harvard University Press.

White, M. (2007). *Maps of narrative practice.* New York: W. W. Norton.

White, M. (2004). Working with people who are suffering the consequences of multiple trauma. *The International Journal of Narrative Therapy and Community Work, 1,* 45-76.

White, M. (1997). *Narratives of therapists' lives.* Adelaide, Australia: Dulwich Centre Publications.

White, M. (1988). Saying hello again: The incorporation of the lost relationship in the resolution of grief, in *Selected Papers,* Dulwich Centre Publications, pp. 29-36.

White, M., & Epston, D. (1990). *Narrative means to therapeutic ends.* New York: Norton.

Young, K. (2008). Narrative practice at a walk-in therapy clinic: Developing children's worry wisdom. *Journal of Systemic Therapies, 27,* 54-74.

Young, K. (2006). *When all the time you have is now: Narrative practice at a walk-in therapy clinic.* Retrieved 07/02/2010 from www.brieftherapynetwork.com/papers.htm.

Young, K., Dick, M., Herring, K., Lee, J. (2008). From waiting lists to walk-in: Stories from a walk-in therapy clinic. *Journal of Systemic Therapies, 27,* 23-39.

Young, K., & Cooper, S. (2008). Toward co-composing an evidence base: The narrative therapy re-visiting project. *Journal of Systemic Therapies, 27,* 67-83.

Chapter 9

From Imagination to Reality: Mental Health Walk-In at South Calgary Health Centre

Sandy Harper-Jaques, RN, MN, RMFT
and *Maureen Leahey, RN, Ph.D.*

Imagine a mental health service where the client or family presents, and after completing two consumer friendly forms, the client is seen for an hour of therapy by a qualified therapist. And, also imagine that this service is offered at no charge to the client. The cost is covered by the client's health insurance. Also consider that the client chooses when the walk-in therapy session will occur. He, she, or they arrive, during the hours that the service is open, without a referral or an appointment. And, imagine that this service is able to see the client, on average, within 20 minutes from the time that the client completes forms. This service is not imaginary; it exists. It is the Mental Health Walk-In Program (MHWI) located in the South Calgary Health Centre (SCHC) in Calgary, Alberta, Canada. The business plan for the centre emphasizes the importance of providing a continuum of community-based services close to people's homes

(Calgary Health Region, 2004). Services include urgent care, laboratory, mental health, community health, medical rehabilitation and management of chronic health concerns (for example: diabetes, respiratory problems and end stage renal disease). The planners also anticipated that these services would reduce the demand for service in hospital emergency rooms.

In this chapter we describe how the MHWI service, which is based on the model developed by Eastside Family Centre described in Chapter 6, operates within a large, publicly funded health care system. The origins of this walk-in service are discussed, followed by a description of the service, the process of therapy and the population served. The theoretical models and philosophies informing the work will be addressed and clinical examples provided. We also address the partnerships and linkages between MHWI and other programs, as well as the methods used to enhance these connections. Effectiveness outcome data are presented. Implications for clients, the larger Alberta Health Services system and training are offered.

Origins

MHWI is an integrated component of SCHC, which is part of Alberta Health Services, a very large provincial organization of over 95,000 employees, delivering a network of health services. In Alberta there is a province-wide framework for the delivery of mental health and addictions services. This framework supports the provision of adequate, easily accessible and integrated care at a level that is most appropriate for the consumer. In response to a significant population growth in the south quadrant of Calgary and concerns regarding the lack of services for this population, Alberta Health Services opened the SCHC in 2004. In addition to a full range of medical services, a continuum of mental health services was created in recognition that "many patients with mental health concerns are currently waiting for treatment at locations that already have long wait lists, are far from their homes and/or are not optimal sites for interventions" (Syverson, 2006, p. v.) These services include Mental Health Walk-In, Mental Health Urgent Care (MHUC), Adult Mental Health, Child/Adolescent Mental Health, Mobile Response Team (MRT) and Community Geriatric Mental Health Service. The services share the same goals:

- To provide easy access to mental health services,
- To develop and maintain practices and partnerships that enhance service coordination and client transition to the most appropriate care,
- To provide services with positive client outcomes,
- To provide learning and development opportunities for staff.

Description of Mental Health Walk-In

The MHWI is open 4-7 PM Monday through Thursday and 12-3 PM on Sundays. These hours were chosen to facilitate access. People can walk in on their way home from work, or when a child is the focus of concern, the child and parent(s) can come after school. The MHWI waiting room is shared with Community Health, Speech and Language and Rehabilitation programs. Three qualified therapists work each walk-in shift. Therapists have graduate degrees, are licensed as a nurse, social worker or psychologist and have many years experience working with mental health issues. Therapists use a variety of theoretical approaches. One of the therapists is assigned the role of shift coordinator. The shift coordinator manages the flow of clients, consults with the therapist and ensures the quality of treatment provided. The shift coordinator and team observe the therapy session from behind a one-way mirror.

The clinical conversation in a MHWI session is different than a conversation in which the therapist and client expect to continue therapy in another session. The therapist works quickly to establish a working alliance and engage the client. Interventive questions (Tomm, 1987; Tomm, 1988) such as Wright's (1989) "one question question" (If there was one question you could have answered during our time together, what would your one question be?) are used to ascertain what the client needs. A collaborative conversation evolves in which the presenting concern is discussed and attempted solutions are explored. (A DSM-IV-TR assessment is not completed.) The therapist listens for both the client's ideas about change and readiness to do something differently. The therapist's theoretical orientation during the interview might be cognitive-behavioral, family systems, narrative, Solution-Focused or a melding of several models. A description of the process of MHWI therapy is outlined in Figure 1.

Even though the service is designed to provide a single-session, clients/families can return to MHWI in the future. In fact, in the 2009-2010 fiscal year, 31% of the clients seen had come to MHWI previously for a single-session of therapy. In most cases, the client/family will see a different therapist. This is for two reasons. One, the Eastside single-session model emphasizes the client's engagement with the service not the therapist; and, secondly, therapists rotate in and out of the service. A particular therapist may not be working the next time the client presents.

Population Served

During the April 1, 2009 to March 31, 2010 fiscal year, MHWI conducted 814 single sessions of therapy with clients of all ages (Alberta Health Services, 2010). This is a 17% increase over 2007-2008. It was the first visit to MHWI

Figure 1. A Description of the Process of MHWI Therapy

1. Client/family presents at the clinic and asks to talk to someone.
2. The admitting clerk registers the client and asks all family members who plan to participate in the session to complete two consumer-friendly forms.
3. The admitting clerk notifies the shift coordinator when the client arrives and when the forms are completed.
4. The team meets to review the forms and generate hypotheses and ideas for the session.
5. The therapist meets with the client/family for 30 – 45 minutes while the team observes through a one-way mirror. Observation and the role of the team are discussed with the client at the beginning of the session.
6. The therapist takes a break and consults the shift coordinator and team.
7. The therapist briefly meets again with the client/family to provide ideas, information and/or tasks.
8. The client/family leave the service.
9. The team debriefs the session; therapist documents the interview.

for 69% of the clients. During this fiscal year, 87% of the clients lived on the south side of the city. During this fiscal year (2009-2010), therapists met with 596 individuals (75%), 80 couples (10 %) and 119 families (15%).

Of the registered clients, 61% were female and 39% male. Since opening in 2004, the majority of our clients have been adults between the ages of 25 and 54. This fiscal year was consistent with that trend; 61% of the registered clients were in this age range. The most frequently cited presenting concerns have also been consistent since 2004. In 2009-2010, the concerns identified by clients were depression (21%) and anxiety (14%). Relationship concerns such as couple, parent-child, family and divorce/separation constituted 17% of the presenting issues. Very few client presentations necessitated a higher level of care. Of the 814 clients seen, 4% were transferred to Mental Health Urgent Care (MHUC) co-located in SCHC and 29% were discharged home with new ideas about how to address their concerns. An additional 25% were given some new ideas and information about community agencies and 25% were invited to seek a referral for mental health services provided through Alberta Health Services.

Theoretical Models and Philosophical Influences

In the early 1990's clinicians such as Slive (Slive, MacLaurin, Oakander & Amundsen, 1995; Slive, McElheran & Lawson, 2008) began to imagine "a whole therapy in an hour," a therapy that had a beginning, middle and end in a single-session. The imagining became the Eastside single-session model described in Chapter 3. This model invites therapists to reconsider ideas about the pace of change and the nature of the therapeutic relationship. Therapists who agree to practice in a single-session therapy program such as MWHI are expected to ascribe to concepts such as: effective help can be provided in one hour to a client the therapist may never see again; clients are the experts in knowing what they need and knowing when to ask for help; and the client's ability to solve problems can be accessed in order to find new solutions. The stance of the therapist is that of consultant to the client (Harper-Jaques, McElheran, Slive & Leahey, 2008). During the session, the story of the client's concerns, the attempted solutions and information about the client's readiness for change evolves. The therapist may (or may not) discover why the client has decided to seek help today. After the therapist and client have talked for about 30 – 45 minutes, the therapist takes a break to consult with the team. During the consultation with the team, the therapist formulates some ideas to offer to the client. The therapist and team endeavor to match these ideas with the perceived needs of the client. The therapist's hope in offering ideas to the client is to provide information in a manner that fits with the client's view of change (Wright & Leahey, 2009). A list of sample interventions developed by MHWI therapists is presented in Figure 2.

Partnerships and Linkages

A review of therapy models reveals the close link between a particular model and the context in which the model was conceived and developed. For example, Minuchin's structural family therapy model was developed in a community center in the slums of Philadelphia with the goal of empowering and healing inner-city families who faced challenges such as poverty and racism. The Milan team's model evolved to provide treatment to families who had failed at resolving their difficulties through conventional therapies. In Part 1 of this book, Slive and Bobele describe the theoretical foundations, conception and evolution of a single-session family therapy model situated in a stand alone community based service. While the MHWI service at SCHC is based on the same theoretical foundations, its implementation and on-going development have been influenced by its context (Harper-Jaques, McElheran, Slive & Leahey, 2008).

Figure 2. **SAMPLE MHWI INTERVENTIONS**

- Bibliotherapy
- Relaxation exercises
- Reading a story to the client at the end of the session.
- Exploring exceptions
- Externalizing the problem
- Taking notes or writing down ideas (a clipboard and pad of paper are kept in the therapy room).
- Asking the client/family to complete a writing assignment during the break.
- Providing a team reflection.
- Acknowledging strengths and offering commendations.
- Linking the client with other SCHC and/or community services.
- Providing a therapeutic letter with the team's reflections about the session.
- Giving the client a paper collage to take away.
- Observation tasks

The SCHC's MHWI is embedded in a continuum of mental health services where attention is paid to both the interface among the various mental health programs and the communication between providers who come from a variety of disciplines such as nursing, social work or psychology. This ecological systems (Auerswald 1968; Auerswald, 1998) approach puts the needs of a particular client or family at the centre, ahead of the epistemology of a particular discipline or the guidelines of a certain model of therapy or mental health program. Discussions within the MHWI team or between therapists from other SCHC mental health programs focus on how the intervention can assist the client.

As noted earlier, one of the goals of the mental health services within SCHC is "to develop and maintain practices and partnerships that enhance service coordination and client transition to the most appropriate care." At SCHC, the ecological systems approach is important in meeting this goal. This approach fosters information exchange and transfer of clients to the mental health service that best fits their needs. The following clinical example from our program that explains our point of view is the story of Seema, age 45. Her main concerns when she presented to MHWI were lack of motivation, frequent crying and frequent absences from work. On the day of her presentation to MHWI her supervisor talked with her about frequent use of sick time and asked her to seek help. The therapist and team offered three concrete ideas for her to use to ensure she went to work. Seema agreed with these ideas but expressed doubt that she would use them because of low motivation. The services of the Mobile Response Team (MRT) were explained to Seema and, with her verbal consent, the MRT was consulted. A decision was made to offer Seema a follow-up call or visit from the MRT. Seema looked relieved and agreed to receive a phone call from the team. A member of the MRT came into the therapy room to meet Seema. A plan was developed for a phone call and the walk-in session ended.

Another example of the SCHC's MHWI focus on service coordination is the attention paid to larger systems. During the presession discussion, the therapist and team considers the client's larger system. This term generally refers to work, school systems, healthcare and providers as well as social agencies such as public welfare or child protection (Wright & Leahey, 2009). Responses to questions on the consumer friendly presession MHWI forms provide the therapist and team with ideas about the client's larger system relationships. During the presession discussion the therapist and team may consider questions such as: who is more interested in the client coming here today, the client or the child welfare worker?; what is the nature of the relationship between this client and her school environment?; how often does this client meet with her physician?; what is the physician's level of concern about the client's emotional health distress? During the session, the therapist may talk with the client about her partnership with larger systems' health providers (Johnson, 2000). This may include the client's desire to involve his physician in providing support for the mental health concern by sending a copy of the MHWI session notes to the family physician.

At times, clients who present to MHWI require immediate medical care, a psychiatric assessment or hospitalization. This occurs about 2 to 3 times each month. In these instances the MHWI service works in a collaborative partnership with the Urgent Care department at South Calgary Health Centre to ensure support and safety of the client (Southern, Leahey, Harper-Jaques, McGonigal & Syverson, 2007; Yonge & Austin, 2010). During the 2009-2010 fiscal year, 4% of clients who presented to MHWI required urgent care. The MHWI therapist provides pertinent verbal and written information to both the triage nurse in Urgent Care and the MHUC nurse in order to facilitate the transfer.

For example, Paul (22) came to MHWI with his girlfriend. Both individuals looked tired and worried at the start of the session. On the presession forms, Paul indicated that his risk of harming himself was moderate. At the beginning of the session, the shift coordinator asked the MHUC nurse to join the team behind the mirror. When the therapist asked about risk, Paul and his girlfriend talked about his previous history of suicidal ideation and attempts. Paul talked about solutions he had tried to manage his current thoughts, but he did not feel that they were working. The young couple expressed worry about Paul's safety. They reported few social or family supports in Calgary. When the therapist consulted with the team and evaluated risk factors, a decision was made to provide this couple with a choice of transfer to Mental Health Urgent Care or follow-up the next day with the MRT. When the options were offered, they both looked relieved when Mental Health Urgent Care was offered. The MHUC nurse joined the session, and escorted the couple to Urgent Care. The MHWI shift coordinator was later told that Paul was admitted to hospital. The client's transfer from one service to another with a minimum of additional "hoop jumping" on the client's part, was seamless.

Another example of this collaborative partnership is the relationship between community health and the mental health programs at SCHC. Studies (O'Hara, Swain, Starr & Gorman, 1997) support universal screening of postpartum women for depression. Veitch and Geake's (2008) evaluation project noted that 13% of postpartum women in Alberta report symptoms of a mood disorder severe enough to require further assessment and intervention. In Calgary, community health nurses watch for signs of depression in the postpartum population. They also administer the Edinburgh postnatal depression scale (Cox, Holden & Sagvosky, 1987) to high-risk women within three to six weeks of delivery or during the mother and baby's two-month visit to the Well Child Clinic. In situations where a woman's score is of concern, the community health nurse refers the woman to mental health. When MHWI is open, the community health nurse at SCHC simply walks the woman across the waiting room (mental health and community health share the same waiting room) and asks that the new mother be seen in MHWI.

Jennifer (29) came to MHWI after a visit in the Well Child Clinic. She had delivered her second baby eight weeks earlier. During the visit in the Well Child Clinic, the nurse noticed Jennifer's monotone voice and her unchanging facial expression. Jennifer cared for her baby during the visit but the care looked "mechanical" and Jennifer did not engage with the baby. The score on the Edinburgh postnatal depression scale indicated that mental health consultation was required. When the nurse offered a session in MHWI, Jennifer agreed. She called her husband, who was at home caring for the couple's 3 year old, and told him of her plan to go the MHWI. After the therapist and team reviewed the MHWI forms Jennifer had completed, the therapist met with Jennifer and her baby. The therapist immediately noted Jennifer's sad facial expression and her blunted affect. Jennifer told the therapist that she did well following the birth of their first child. She was aware that things were different this time. She was crying a lot; she had little energy and she did not enjoy caring for this baby like she had for her first baby. Recently, Jennifer had stopped visiting with other at-home moms in her neighbourhood, and she no longer attended a support group at her church. When the therapist asked about thoughts of suicide, Jennifer started to weep; she told the therapist she was scared by the thoughts she had about ending her life. She said she did not have a plan and she would not hurt her children. Jennifer looked relieved when the therapist told her help was available. The therapist consulted with the team and weighed the risk and protective factors; they decided the protective factors outweighed the risks. The team wanted to increase support to Jennifer and her family. With Jennifer's permission, the therapist called Jennifer's husband and asked him to come to MHWI to join the session. When he arrived, the therapist provided the couple with information about postpartum depression. With the therapist's help, the couple devised a plan to ensure Jennifer's safety at home. The therapist also offered the resources of the MRT and quick access to therapy at the AMH program at SCHC. The couple was also referred to a community-based program for families with newborns, and Jennifer was encouraged to make an appointment with her family doctor. When the therapist's notes were completed, copies were sent to the community health nurse, the family physician and the therapist who would be contacting Jennifer from the AMH program.

Using MHWI for waitlist management is another example of a practice that enhances client transition to the most appropriate level of care. In a publicly funded health system such as the Alberta Health Services, demand often outpaces available resources. MHWI is one way of providing immediate service to people while they are waiting to enter on-going outpatient therapy. Clients referred to the SCHC Adult Mental Health or Child/Adolescent Programs are provided with information about MHWI when their names are placed on the program's waiting list. For example, a person who is placed on the Adult Mental Health program waiting list for treatment of panic disorder may present to MHWI seeking a few ideas of ways to cope or manage panic attacks. These programs can then obtain notes from the walk-in session when the client is registered in their program.

Methods to Enhance Linkages and Continuity of Care

To achieve the goals of MHWI, various methods and organizational processes have been instituted to enhance linkages and facilitate continuity of care.

Staffing

Therapists who work in MHWI are either regularly scheduled to work in the service or they are called in to work on an as-needed basis. The regularly scheduled therapists also work in other SCHC mental health programs. This arrangement improves efficiency because therapists complete clinical paper-work associated with their role in the other program during walk-in down time. Each of the AMH therapists works one walk-in shift per week and one Sunday shift every four weeks. The Child/Adolescent Mental Health program provides a part-time therapist to MHWI. The child and adolescent therapists have specialized knowledge and expertise about therapy with clients who are under the age of 18. Having this expertise on the team is very important as there are a large number of families with children and adolescents living in the south end of the city. Some of the MHWI relief staff work in other Alberta Health Services mental health programs. This fosters the infusion of ideas about single-session therapy into other areas of practice. The combination of therapists who work in different programs promotes ease of transfer of clients from one service to another.

Therapists work as a team. Every therapist/discipline participates on the team as an observer, a therapist, a consultant and at times, as a shift coordinator. (The shift coordinator role is assigned on a rotating basis to the therapists who regularly work in MHWI.) Every discipline assumes a leadership role and all therapists are invited and expected to contribute ideas regarding the client's presentation. Among the team members there is a culture of respect for each other and for the client. This culture of respect includes some unwritten rules: such as no criticism of the treating therapists by observing therapists and no criticism or judgmental comments about clients by therapists who are observing. When disagreements occur among the team members, the discussion is focused on the issue, not on the therapist's personal characteristics.

Administrative Structure

Since the MHWI program opened, a number of procedures and structures have been developed to support our clients and the therapists. These procedures facilitate client transfer and information exchange from one program/service to another. This not only eliminates "hoop jumping" on the part of the client, it reduces the amount of information the client has to re-tell another health care provider. The clinical supervisor for MHWI is also clinical supervisor for AMH and a consultant to MHUC. Similar to other team members, the supervisor works one walk-in shift per week and one Sunday shift every four weeks. She also takes turns as a shift coordinator. There are several regularly scheduled meetings intended to foster relationships within or between different services. These include regular business meetings with the shift coordinators, whole team discussions focused on clinical challenges and dilemmas and semi-annual meetings with team members from both MHUC and AMH. Examples of the clinical vignettes discussed in the MHWI whole team discussions are included in Appendix B.

Shared space is another mechanism for increasing linkages among staff and fostering continuity of care. Several of the SCHC programs (MHWI, Adult Mental Health, Mobile Response Team, Community Geriatric Mental Health and Child/Adolescent Mental Health) are co-located in cubicles in the same open office area. In addition to sharing the same workspace, they share therapy rooms, secretarial support and office equipment. This has fostered mutual support and an understanding of the operations and challenges among the teams.

DOCUMENTATION

After the end of the session, the therapist writes a brief note about the client's session in MHWI. Risk factors, presenting concerns, interventions offered and client responses are all documented. The note is saved in both paper and electronic formats. The paper copy of the client's MHWI note is placed on the client's main service chart and stored in the SCHC Health Records department. This insures that information about the single-session of therapy is available to other health care providers in SCHC on an as-needed basis. The electronic note is placed on a secure shared drive. This permits other mental health providers in Alberta Health Services emergency rooms and Urgent Care centres to follow up on the recommendations and interventions that MHWI offered to the client.

EDUCATION OF STUDENTS

Since it opened, the MHWI has provided observational experiences and practicum placements for students from nursing, social work and psychology. The variety of client concerns, the opportunity to observe therapists from different disciplines and therapeutic orientations and the experience of participating in a multidisciplinary team provide students with a rich learning environment. Students who observe MHWI tend to be undergraduate students interested in learning more about the delivery of mental health care. They are provided with a small packet of information about MHWI and asked to read an article prior to joining the team. Practicum students are masters or Ph.D. students who will use their clinical experience in MHWI as a portion of their practicum hours. These students are oriented to MHWI by first participating in a three-hour seminar about the model and practice of single-session therapy at SCHC. As follow-up to the seminar they are encouraged to read about single-session therapy. They are also expected to join the walk-in team, as an observer for two shifts when their clinical supervisor is working MHWI. At the end of this orientation process, the clinical supervisor and student determine if the student is ready to meet with clients who present to walk-in.

Having students aware of MHWI has benefitted patient care. These students spread the word about the quick access and quality of service. As they moved from one student placement to another, they have become ambassadors for the program.

EFFECTIVENESS

There has been considerable interest in the effectiveness of the service. Syverson (2006) reported on an evaluation of MHWI conducted between May and October 2005. Evaluation goals were:

1. To determine whether MHWI was associated with easy access to mental health care,
2. To provide information regarding client transition and service coordination/collaborative partnerships,
3. To determine whether clients using MHWI have desirable outcomes and are satisfied with various aspects of the service received.

To address these goals, several methods were used including manual and electronic data systems, interviews or focus groups and client written self-report questionnaires.

Results regarding Goal #1 (ease of access) showed that 65% of clients (n=154) were seen within 30 minutes or less from the time they presented to the admitting clerk; clients were seen, on average, within 13 minutes of handing in their completed intake questionnaires. The average session lasted about an hour. Twenty-seven percent of clients indicated previous mental health involvement during the previous year. If the MHWI were not open, 70% of clients indicated they would have sought service elsewhere for their mental health concerns. Alternate service choices included acute care hospital (8%), general practitioner/medical walk-in clinic (22%), addiction services (6%) and psychiatrist/psychologist (4%).

Findings relating to Goal #2 (client transition and collaborative partnerships) showed that upon discharge from MHWI, 62% of clients were provided with service and/or psychoeducational material while 20% were referred to other SCHC mental health services. Interestingly, of the clients seen in MHUC (n= 438) 23% of the referrals from MHUC were sent to MHWI. This was a very positive finding because MHWI is an interventive program and most appropriate for these clients to access in future times of distress.

Results pertaining to Goal # 3 (desirable client outcomes and satisfaction) indicated clients (n=188) reported a mean presession distress level of 7.9

and a postsession mean of 5.4 on a ten-point scale. Paired samples t-tests were used and a statistically significant difference was noted with clients experiencing a drop in distress. Satisfaction results indicated clients (n=150) were satisfied or delighted with:

- Ability of staff to listen and understand your problems (97%)
- How involved and caring the staff is (95%)
- Knowledge and skills of the staff (94%)

Aspects of MHWI that clients liked the least included:

- The time limit and/or single-session nature of the appointment (n=7)
- The problem wasn't completely resolved (n=14)

Following up on Syverson's report, we conducted evaluation studies in MHWI from April 2006 through March 31, 2007. MHWI clients (n=317) reported a mean presession distress level of 8.18 and a postsession mean of 5.45, a statistically significant difference, A paired samples t-test was used to analyze the data. Once again, MHWI client outcomes were very positive. Clients experienced a significant drop in distress.

Client satisfaction data is available for 7 months of 2007. Of the 240 clients who answered a written questionnaire about overall satisfaction with the service, 94% stated they were satisfied or delighted. Clients were 91% satisfied or delighted regarding the therapist's knowledge and skills, ability to listen, understand and care. Clients were also satisfied or delighted with the:

- Accessibility and location of the service (89%, n=244),
- Hours the service is open (80%, n= 244),
- Ability to access the service without a referral (98%, n=226),
- Time they waited to be seen (83%, n=245).

The satisfaction results were consistent with Syverson's (2006) earlier findings.

From April through September 2009, clients (n=196) were asked "If MHWI didn't exist, where would you go for service?" Again, the findings are consistent with the 2006 results with 14% stating they would have gone to a hospital/acute care site, 10% to a family doctor's office and 13% to a counseling agency. Having MHWI services provided and accessible in a community health centre is much less expensive than service in a hospital or a physician's office.

One area of concern from Syverson's (2006) initial evaluation was low client satisfaction ratings with family involvement in sessions. Of the clients (n=150) surveyed in 2005, only 78% were satisfied/delighted with "the extent to which your family/significant other(s) were involved in your care". The low rating was disquieting to both therapists and management. A follow-up evaluation was undertaken from September 2007 through February 2008 to increase understanding in two areas: first, how clients want their family/friends involved in care and second, client and family/friend satisfaction with the current involvement (Foucault, Harper-Jaques, Leahey & Southern, 2009). The 179 MHWI clients were divided into three groups: Group 1 clients (n=49) with family in session; Group 2 clients (n=30) with family in waiting room; and Group 3 clients (n=100) seen alone.

The 179 clients and 64 family/friends completed brief written self-report ratings and open-ended questionnaires. Overall, 86% of clients who had a family member/friend participate in the session felt the family/friend was sufficiently involved with all dimensions of care. When clients in this group reported low satisfaction with family/friend involvement, it was primarily because they wanted their family/friends to be more active in sharing information or concerns that they felt were important, providing their opinion about how the client was doing and receiving practical advice on how to cope with the situation.

Often, if family/friends did not join clients in the session it was not both their preferences. Of the 30 clients who had family/friend in the waiting room, 43% of clients stated they wanted the person in the waiting room to join them and 13% of family/friends who were waiting had hoped to attend the session. Among clients (n=100) who came to MHWI alone, 34% would have preferred to have a family member or friend join them.

These findings were shared with the therapists who work in MHWI. They confirmed the therapists' views about clients' interpersonal connectedness. In response to these findings three changes were made in the MHWI program. The first change involved the addition of two questions on the pre-session forms about whether the client came alone or with someone. Clients were asked if the person who came with them to MHWI would participate in the session. This question was meant to stimulate an awareness of interpersonal connections and to respect client wishes about who would be involved in the session. The second change was the placement of clipboards, paper and pencil in the MHWI therapy rooms. During the break near the end of the session, clients who come alone are encouraged to use the paper to write notes about the session to share with a family member or friend. The third change was MHWI therapists developed questions to use when involving family members in the therapeutic conversation.* This was to ensure that family members who

* Questions to ask family/friends who come into the walk-in therapy session…

- At the outset of the session, when family and friends are present it is useful to clarify roles, the expectations about the level of involvement of the family member or friend.
- Questions to family members could include: "what is your hope/goal for today's session?", how do you understand the issue/problem?", what solutions have been tried?"
- The questions asked of the family members/friends – "how do you think you can be helpful/involved in today's session?"

attended sessions were included in the therapy. The questions also helped clinicians remember that, because family/friends may be less familiar with the client's mental health concerns, they will likely require more information about the client's presenting problem, possible interventions and coping strategies.

Along with the family involvement survey, clients also completed pre and postsession distress ratings in 2007-2008. Once again, there was a significant decrease in distress levels using paired samples t-tests (p>001). Clients seen with family/friend n=44, had pre-mean 7.91 and post-mean 5.1; clients with family/friend in waiting room n=27, had a pre-mean 8.04 and post-mean 4.96; clients seen alone n=96 had a pre-mean 7.78, and post-mean 5.2.

Implications

There are several implications of having a MHWI service in SCHC. For clients, there is timely access for a high quality service easily available with no appointment and no referral. Having this mental health service available may prevent exacerbation of the mental health problem and resulting need for more extensive services.

Implications for Alberta Health Services are that it reduces the use of mental health services in acute care sites that are designed to serve people with higher acuity. This is a cost savings for Alberta Health Services and provides a more effective treatment to consumer. MHWI is an intervention resource, not merely an assessment service. Using staff from various Alberta Health Services programs promotes the walk-in model within the organization and fosters brief therapeutic conversation with clients.

For students, the opportunity to participate in collaborative interdisciplinary clinical teams is a valuable learning experience. There is a rich exchange of ideas about clinical problems and interventions. MHWI provides a venue for student supervision with its one-way mirrors, video and strong teamwork.

Conclusions

A framework for the delivery of Addiction and Mental Health services has been developed by Alberta Health Services. MHWI is a vital component of the framework (Alberta Health Services, 2009). It delivers consistent service in a timely manner, increases linkages and facilitates transfer of clients when more intensive service is required. It is a strength based, collaborative, accessible, client-centered service. Located in the community, it is aligned with community based resources as well as Alberta Health Services programs. Therapists evaluate risk and protective factors and are accountable for their evidence-informed practice. The MHWI service philosophy is fundamentally rooted in a bio-psychosocial-spiritual and cultural perspective valuing a range of approaches offered by diverse disciplines. It has a place in the universal and targeted prevention and health promotion part of an integrated service delivery framework. It also moves beyond prevention by offering brief timely intervention to clients seeking assistance.

The saying "it take a village to raise a child" can apply equally in offering SCHC MHWI. The collaboration of interdisciplinary staff, management and students is essential in delivering quality service to clients. We are privileged to be part of this.

The authors wish to acknowledge the dedicated and creative work of the walk-in therapists who were working with us when we wrote this chapter. Their names are: Monica Barnes, RN, MN, Susan Brown, BA, MSW, RSW, Pat Carruthers, RPN, PhD, Teresa Coker, MSW, RSW, Darlene Foucault, PhD ,R. Psych, Tanya Hofer, MSW, RSW, Pamela Klein, MSW, RSW, Adrienne Krentz, MSc, R. Psych, Lisa-Jo Leslie, MSW, RSW, Angela Lounsberry, BA, MSW, RSW, Amy Marshall, RN, MN, Bev Nackoney, RPN, MC, R. Psych (Prov.), Maureen Osis, RN, MN, Maja Popovic, MSc., R. Psych, Caroline Schnitzler, PhD, R. Psych, Janet Wilson, MEd, R. Psych, Lesa Wolfe, PhD, RSW, Susan Young, MA, R. Psych.

References

Alberta Health Services. (2010). *Mental Health and Addictions Walk-In Annual Report, 2009-2010* Unpublished document.

Alberta Health Services. (2009). *Mental health and addiction integrated service delivery framework.* Progress update, February 18, 2009. Unpublished document.

Auerswald, E. H. (1968). Interdisciplinary versus ecological approach. *Family Process, 7,* 202-215.

Auerswald, E. H. (1998). Interdisciplinary versus ecological approach. *Families, Systems & Health 16,* 299-308.

Calgary Health Region (2004). *Business Case – South Link Mental Health Growth.* Unpublished report. Calgary Health Region, Calgary, Alberta, Canada.

Cox, J. L., Holden, J. M. & Sagvosky, R. (1987). Edinburgh post-natal depression scale (EPDS). *British Journal of Psychiatry, 150,* 782-786.

Foucault, D., Harper-Jaques, S., Leahey, M. & Southern, L. (2009). *Perceptions of family involvement in mental health care: Through the lens of clients and their families.* Poster presented at 9th International Family Nursing Conference, Reykjavik, Iceland June 2- 5, 2009.

Harper-Jaques, S. McElheran, N. Slive, A. & Leahey, M. (2008). A comparison of two approaches to the delivery of walk-in single session mental health therapy. *Journal of Systemic Therapies, 27*(4), 40-53.

Johnson, B. M. (2000). Family-centered care: Four decades of progress. *Families, Systems & Health, 18* (2), 137-156.

O'Hara, A.M., Swain, M.W., Starr, K.R., & Gorman, L.L. (1997). A prospective study of sleep, mood, and cognitive function in postpartum women. *Obstetrics and Gynecology, 90* (3), 381-386.

Miller, J. & Slive, A. (2004). Breaking down the barriers to clinical service delivery: Walk-In family therapy. *Journal of Marital and Family Therapy, 30,* 95-103.

Slive, A. , McElheran, N. & Lawson, A. (2008). How brief does it get? Walk-In single session therapy. *Journal of Systemic Therapies, 27* (4), 5-22.

Slive, A. MacLaurin, B, Oakander, M, & Amundsen, J. (1995). Walk-in single sessions: A new paradigm in clinical service delivery. *Journal of Systemic Therapies, 14* (1), 3-11.

Southern, L., Leahey, M., Harper-Jaques, S., McGonigal, K. & Syverson, A. (2007). Integrating mental health into urgent care in a community health centre. *Canadian Nurse, 103* (1), 29-34.

Syverson, A. (2006). *Final report: South Calgary Health Centre – New Mental Health Services Evaluation.* Unpublished Report. Calgary Health Region, Calgary, Alberta, Canada.

Tomm, K. (1987). Interventive interviewing: Part II. Reflexive questioning as a means to enable self-healing. *Family Process, 26,* 167-183.

Tomm, K. (1988). Interventive interviewing: Part III. Intending to ask linear, circular, strategic or reflexive questions? *Family Process, 27,* 1-15.

Veitch, T & Geake, C. (2008). *Postpartum depression project evaluation report.* Unpublished Report. Calgary Health Region, Calgary, Alberta, Canada.

Wright, L. M. (1989). When clients ask questions: Enriching the therapeutic conversation. *Family Therapy Networker, 13 (*6), 15-16.

Wright, L. M. & Leahey, M. (2009). *Nurses and families: A guide to family assessment and intervention.* (5th ed). Philadelphia: F. A. Davis.

Yonge, O., & Austin, W. (2010). Contemporary psychiatric and mental health nursing practice. (pp. 71-81). In Austin, W. & Boyd, M. A. (eds). *Psychiatric nursing for Canadian practice.* Philadelphia. Lippincott, Williams & Wilkins.

Chapter 10

Single-Session Intervention in the Wake of Hurricane Katrina: Strategies for Disaster Mental Health Counseling

John K. Miller, Ph.D., LMFT

What is needed is for our most basic assumptions in psychological thought to be revised from the bottom up. But this revision cannot be made from our offices.
—Ignacio Martín-Baró

Hurricane Katrina

Hurricane Katrina formed in the Bahamas on August 23, 2005, crossing Florida before strengthening in the Gulf of Mexico and making a second landfall in southeast Louisiana on the morning of August 29. It was the costliest hurricane in American history, and among the five deadliest in recorded history. The storm is estimated to have caused over $100 billion in damage. Hardest hit of the southern states was Louisiana, where flooding from the storm surge caused a catastrophic failure of the levee system. Ultimately 80% of the New Orleans area would flood, as well as many neighboring parishes. Boats, barges, and cars were pushed as far as 12 miles inland, ramming buildings and causing more damage to the levee system. High winds felled scores of large trees, destroying homes, cutting power lines, and blocking roadways. Weeks after the storm many people in affected areas were still living without power, water, phones, or basic supplies. Four years after the storm thousands of residents were still living in temporary trailers. Over 1,836 people lost their lives in the hurricane and subsequent floods.

Shortly after the storm, the American Red Cross sent hundreds of Disaster Mental Health (DMH) workers to the southern states to provide emergency counseling services to the survivors (Miller, 2006). Most of the counseling that occurred involved a walk-in (or walk-up) single-session meeting. This chapter describes some of the counseling work that was carried out after the storm, with specific attention to the principles of single-session therapy relevant to DMH counseling.

Origins of My Walk-In Single-Session Work

My history with walk-in single-session therapy began in 1995 when I moved from the US to Canada to join the therapy staff of the Eastside Therapy Center (EFC) in Calgary (Chapter 6) as part of my-year long doctoral internship in marriage and family therapy. I chose this site to complete my clinical internship because of the pioneering work being done at the center offering a walk-in, single-session as one of the primary modes of clinical service delivery. I had read about the unique service at the Eastside Centre in a groundbreaking article published that year (Slive, MacLaurin, Oakander, & Amundson, 1995). As a brief therapist, I was intrigued by this briefest of therapies.

I was skeptical about how useful a single-session could really be, but after watching and participating in the service I quickly realized that something special was happening at the EFC. The therapy done at the clinic was exciting and appeared to be very effective for some client situations. Later I decided to do my dissertation study on the client experiences with this therapy and found that 82% of the clients were satisfied. The majority of those who came for a session reported that they were helped. More than half felt the single-session was sufficient to address their concerns and that no further therapy was needed (Miller, 1996; Miller, 2008). For many of the clients, this was their first time to see a therapist. During follow-up interviews I did with 43 clients in a later study, many told me that they would never have considered going to more traditional outpatient therapy services (Miller & Slive, 2004). They came to the EFC because they felt the walk-in single-session intervention was hassle-free, convenient, and especially appealing because the ability to come in at the moment of need.

One of the most compelling aspects of this therapy was that it seemed to attract a group of clients who would likely benefit from services but would have been unlikely to access them. Like most therapists, I had worked with many couples and families in traditional outpatient services who had lived with their problems for years, letting them grow and fester before reaching such painful levels that they would overcome their fear of stigma and shame to actually schedule a session. The landmark US Surgeon General's report on mental health issues in the America revealed that, at some point during their lives, about half of the population of the US will experience a situation where they would likely be helped by accessing mental health services. Further, the report indicated that more than half of the people who would benefit from mental health services would never access them because of barriers to clinical service delivery. The three main barriers to service include stigma, accessibility, and cost (U.S. Department of Health and Human Services, 1999; Murray & Lopez, 1996; Rice & Miller, 1996).

After studying the problem of clinical service delivery, I wondered how much more effective therapy would be if clients would come in for treatment when the problem first emerged. Additionally, much of the therapy I had seen in the US was geared to the middle and upper classes. I felt therapy was viewed by the public as an elitist service that only the well-heeled could afford. I was interested in delivery systems that could overcome those barriers to service. The low-cost, non-stigmatizing emphasis of the walk-in services at the Eastside Family Center presented one ideal solution (Slive et. al, 1995; Bobele, Miller & Slive, 2009; Hoffart & Hoffart, 1994; Miller, 2008; Miller, Banks, Goodwin, Fick, Froerer, & Stroyman, 2006; Miller & Slive, 2004; Miller & Slive, 1997; Miller, 1996; Slive, McElheran, & Lawson, 2002). During my work at the EFC I witnessed many examples of how therapists can make the most of a single-session in therapy. The lessons I learned were that, in many situations, it was possible to promote a lasting change in a single-session intervention, and that one of the most important factors in the process was addressing clients' problems at the moment of need.

I grew up in Louisiana, and began my counseling career in the bayou state in the late 1980's working with underprivileged youth. In the 1990s I was trained by the American Red Cross in Disaster Mental Health (DMH) counseling, with a specific focus on the ideas and techniques of what is commonly called "psychological first aid" (www.redcross.org). So when the call went out from the American Red Cross to serve as a first responder to those impacted by Hurricane Katrina, I enlisted. I completed a typical 2-week tour of duty in and around the New Orleans area providing counseling services to the survivors of the storm and supervision to other DMH workers. Before traveling to the disaster area I participated in a Red Cross conference call that provided a briefing regarding current information about the disaster area, how to prepare for the trip, and what to expect during my deployment. The Red Cross briefer advised DMH workers to prepare for "extreme physical and mental hardship" during the deployment, given reports coming out of the area.

The following describes some of my experiences providing DMH services in the wake of the storm. Almost all the counseling conversations I carried out were via single-session meetings/interventions. I found that much of what I had learned from my experience at the Eastside Family Center was applicable in this new setting.

Theoretical Underpinnings of Single-Session Disaster Mental Health and Strategies for Intervention

Therapy Begins at the First Moment of Meeting

This book details many of the theoretical concepts that are common in the practice of single-session therapy in a variety of settings. Some of these theoretical underpinnings and techniques proved especially useful and relevant for the DMH setting. One of the focal points of a single-session treatment philosophy is making the most of the time you have with clients. In more traditional single-session intervention services, which have developed over the past several decades, this has involved designing the reception, waiting area, and initial paperwork procedures, to be as time efficient as possible. This principle is true in a disaster mental health setting as well.

On my second day in Louisiana I traveled to the New Orleans area and witnessed some of the destruction that had occurred as a result of the storm and the floods that followed. Eventually I was stationed in one of the small towns north of New Orleans, across Lake Pontchartrain where many of the storm refugees fled and were being temporarily housed in Red Cross shelters. Our mission was fairly simple: assist in the shelter and feeding operations, disseminate accurate information, and provide counseling to those who walked in or walked up, whenever possible. There were few private office spaces available. Many people (including the workers) were living in tents, sometimes located on the highway medians. The area was still without electricity or water, so much of the immediate work to be done involved getting people basic supplies, food, and water. To accomplish this the Red Cross teamed up with local churches, agencies, and other volunteer organizations to establish kitchen complexes where people could come each day for a hot lunch and dinner. For those who were homebound, DMH workers traveled in Emergency Response Vehicles (ERVs) that roughly resembled a cross between an ambulance and a delivery truck. The ERVs delivered thousands of boxed hot meals each day by visiting neighborhoods and common areas throughout the affected region. The DMH workers split their time between the kitchen complex, the shelters, and riding along on the ERVs to help deliver food. The basic strategy for the DMH workers was to assist with basic needs while also positioning themselves in places where people with counseling needs would likely visit. This was an effective strategy. About 1 in 20 people who came seeking food and supplies also showed signs of various trauma responses, and would usually readily engage with the DMH workers. Counseling in this context is remarkably different than traditional clinical services. There is no office, no physical trappings of clinical work, and almost invariably the entire therapy was this single meeting.

First Question

Over the last decade the therapists at walk-in single-session services have experimented with various "first questions" for the therapists to ask early in the session to help promote a solvable framing for the problem and the greatest efficiency in a 50-minute session (Miller, 2008; Slive, McElheran, & Lawson, 2002). The following questions, common in brief and solution focused approaches, have proven to be useful in that they do not focus solely on the problem, but on what pragmatically will work for the clients. These questions are useful in that they orient the therapist and the client toward a solvable framing of the problem with a clear direction to proceed. These questions can be modified for DMH work.

What is the single most important concern that you have right now?

This was perhaps the most important organizing question for the DMH counselor to ask. The client's range of needs was great. Some were looking for someone to talk with about a family member or neighbor who was in need of counseling, but they did not know where to turn. Some were dealing with grief and stress that the quick and massive migration from the storm area had brought. Others were looking for someone to talk with because they had lost a family member in the storm, or couldn't find members of their family and feared that they had not survived. Some people were simply dealing with the sudden stop to their lives that had occurred after the storm, because all businesses, services, and social events had ceased.

Depending on the client situation, the therapist had to judge what was the most important type of help that was needed, and prioritize needs (i.e. triage). Focus had to be kept on addressing the most immediate and critical needs first, while keeping the other needs in mind. Some clients needed to be connected with physical resources, such as food and shelter services. Others benefitted more from connecting with family members and the information networks that were established to locate displaced people. To be most effective as a DMH worker, it was important to maintain accurate information about various services, supports, and agencies that could help clients with their physical needs.

The information about these resources changed hourly as new resources became available and others run out. There were multiple agencies converging to provide help, some with overlapping needs or mutual support networks (i.e. one agency has supplies, the other has the capacity to deliver them). Often, one or two seasoned Red Cross workers or other agency workers had a wealth of experience and was current on the ever-changing information about what resources are available. I quickly learned to connect with these seasoned workers and keep a notebook of resource lists that I updated frequently.

WHAT THINGS HAVE YOU TRIED?

This is a typical question in brief therapy, but it takes on new significance in the DMH setting. Naturally, it helps to know what clients have already tried, to avoid doing more of something that is not working. But more than this, it reacquaints the clients with what they've learned about themselves—their existing strength and resources—from past trauma or loss. It can also be a source of encouragement for them to continue with efforts they've already begun to implement. Further, it allows clients to see their strength—their personal approach—as a source of hope, in and of itself. It allows clients to be an integral part in their own healing process.

WHAT INNER STRENGTHS WOULD IT BE USEFUL FOR US TO KNOW ABOUT?

The studies of *resilience* in people after they have experienced a trauma tell us that there are several key factors that tend to promote positive healing and change. One is strong family relationships that foster the ability to develop shared meanings of difficult events shape the foundation of resilience. Other factors include a positive outlook, spiritual convictions, a sense of hope, a feeling of personal control, creativity, and even the ability to utilize humor (Walsh, 2006). Exploring these resiliency factors can be a powerful intervention in helping people begin the process of putting their lives back together in the wake of a disaster.

WHAT WILL BE THE SMALLEST CHANGE TO SHOW YOU THAT THINGS ARE HEADING IN THE RIGHT DIRECTION?

A core initial step in many psychotherapy models (i.e. strategic therapy, cognitive behavioral therapy, solution focused therapy, etc.) includes the process of helping the clients identify and prioritize problems and goals. When there are many problems or goals, the prospect of dealing with them can feel overwhelming for the client. By asking this question in a DMH single-session, you help the client sort out the chaos of the situation they may be experiencing. Breaking the issue down further by focusing on what step can be taken even in this one meeting can give the client some sense of control of the situation that otherwise feels out of control. The job of the therapist in helping the client manage this issue often involves thinking smaller, rather than bigger. As the popular quote by Confucius goes, "the journey of a thousand miles begins with a single step." In DMH figuring out what this first step will be can be the most important step of all.

Pragmatics versus a Specific Model of Intervention

Although each of the DMH workers had their own approach, model, and style for doing therapy, when possible, the counselors worked in pairs as a tteam. This promoted safety and collaboration. Although no one model of therapy is employed in the disaster situation, many of the therapists who provided services tended to use some components of solution focused or brief therapy techniques. In what has become tradition in most single-session approaches, one fundamental goal of the service was to provide clients a clearly identifiable outcome at the end of each session. This outcome was often small and guided by the client's stated goal. To accomplish this in a single session, actions and beliefs needed to be judged by their practical results (Amundson, 1996). Results were evaluated based on whether the session was able to meet the client's stated goal, not on whether the problem was solved. In a DMH setting, the goal was not to resolve the problem, but to help clients have a safe place to talk about loss (if they choose) and deal with the range of feelings and difficulties that were currently present.

It may have been tempting for some therapists to go in directions that might be more typical in outpatient practices. Adjusting to a more pragmatic approach was challenging for some DMH therapists, but it is essential to be most effective in the limited time available. Adjusting to an attitude of pragmatism sometimes challenged the more sacred and deeply felt beliefs about what therapy is and how best to provide it. Those who were successful, however, chose to provide a clear orienting message at the beginning of the meeting (Miller & Slive, 2004). A typical orienting message (in addition to confidentiality/duty to warn and consent discussions) might be as follows:

"Before we begin, I would like to take a minute to explain how we work. As you know, this is a volunteer counseling service; you can come as you have whenever we are available and there is no fee or obligation to return. My hope today is that we can work together in the time that we have (usually about 50 minutes) to help sort things out. You are welcome to return for further counseling any time that we are available, and although you may not be able to meet with me, another DMH worker here will be glad to talk with you."

More is not Better - Better is Better

Therapists at many walk-in single-session centers have adopted a consumer-driven view of how to proceed in therapy. An oversimplified way to put it is that the job of the therapist is to find out what the client wants, and give it to them. From this perspective, therapists avoid second-guessing the client's stated goal by looking for underlying pathology or root problems only. Instead, the therapist approaches the client as a consultant, organized by what the client wants. Often it is difficult for clients to state their wants clearly and requires some processing early in the session. The therapist's task is to guide this process; paying special attention to avoid providing more help than is requested. For example, a client may not be looking for a solution, but simply for someone to talk with.

Naturally, there are exceptions to this approach. It is important to note that in certain situations the therapist must guided first by the ethic of "do not harm." When a child or some other vulnerable client is at risk or there is a risk of self harm or harm to others, the appropriate action is taken (Miller, 2008). The therapist reviews informed consent for treatment and research at the beginning of the session. This includes a description of the limits of confidentiality and the services provided.

But even this necessary intervention is not without problems.

One classic example of sometimes providing more help than is necessary can be seen in the use of the Critical Incident Stress Debriefing (CISD) in DMH situations (Kagee, 2002). This intervention for trauma and accident victims was developed in the 1980's and is still widely used. Yet several recent studies have offered evidence that this intervention often does not work, or does more harm than good with accident victims (Jacobs, Horne-Moyer & Jones, 2004; Mitchelle, Sakraida, & Kameg, 2003). One possible explanation for this surprising finding is that the intervention may provide more help than is needed (or requested).

Timing is Important

In traditional walk-in single-session therapy formats the timing of the clinical delivery is unique because clients chose the time that they wish to access services. The advantage of this situation is that it captures clients' motivational readiness for change (Prochaska & DiClemente, 1992; Hubble, Duncan, & Miller, 1999). One theory about this arrangement is that changes typically sought in therapy are more likely to occur if the counseling is provided at times when there is sufficient motivation and intensity regarding the problem situation (Berg, 1989; Minuchin & Fishman, 1981; deShazer, 1988). Yet in a DMH setting, the goal is somewhat different from other forms of therapy. The goal is not typical problem resolution but helping the clients adjust and deal with the range of new needs and emotions that emerge from the trauma. However, elements of the typical walk-in single-session focus on timing are relevant for DMH work. In disaster situations, providing help at the moment of need is critical. For DMH workers, a focus on timing is enhanced by workers positioning themselves in places where those in need will likely come at those moments when they need help. In the response to Hurricane Katrina the DMH counselors often would work with the other aid personnel to help with delivering food, supplies, and medical care. In this way, they could assist the other helpers to provide for essential needs and also be available at times when the need for counseling services was apparent. In this arrangement the DMH worker was also made aware of the complexities of the other aid duties and tasks. This was sometimes helpful when providing counseling to the other aid workers (i.e. medical services personnel, food supply workers, rescue officers, etc.).

Relationship with the Service versus an Individual Therapist

One disadvantage of a walk-in approach is that it is unlikely that a returning client would be able to see the same therapist should they return for another walk-in session (Miller & Slive, 2004). Given this reality, the philosophy of many walk-in services focuses on promoting a relationship between the client and the service, not the specific individual therapist who provided help. This is even more important in an emergency situation. In a DMH setting, workers often serve only a 2-week tour of duty in the disaster area. Ideally, there is some overlap between the tour of incoming DMH workers and outgoing workers to facilitate a smooth transition. When possible the transition can be facilitated by having incoming DMH workers shadow DMH workers who have been working in the area so they can meet some of the members of the community who may come for help. While most clients are only seen once for counseling, some will return for additional support. After Katrina, the overlap was often limited, so it was important at the end of the session to inform clients that they may not be able to see you again. We would reassure clients that another DMH worker will likely be available, that other DMH workers will welcome the chance to talk, and that people can return as often as they want. The goal here was to help clients develop a relationship with the DMH service in general.

Case Examples: Intervention and Healing

One of the most gratifying experiences for me was to witness, again and again, the open generosity of the citizens of the surrounding communities and their selflessness in helping both those fleeing the storm and those who came to help. The natural resilience of these communities and their members was amazing to witness. In this environment DMH intervention often involved helping catalyze these resiliencies as people worked to get their lives back on track. I offer several examples of the type of work to clarify the implementation of single-session strategies in DMH settings. These examples are drawn from actual experiences, but have been modified to conceal the identities of the clients and the workers involved. In some situations the example is a collection of several different cases merged together to make clear the concepts that are discussed.

Case Example #1: Making a New Home

A senior married couple from the lower 9th ward of New Orleans moved to a shelter north of the area shortly before the storm made landfall. They were referred to the DMH worker by the shelter manager, to help them find a new place to live. The couple had been living at the shelter for over 3 weeks by the time they met with the DMH worker. Their home had been completely destroyed by the storm and the subsequent flood. They only had the two pieces of luggage they had managed to bring with them. Most of the other early refugees at the shelter (those who arrived just after the storm) had by then been connected with family or other supports in other parts of the country and had moved out. However, this couple neither seemed ready to leave the shelter, nor felt very happy about staying.

The shelter environments in Louisiana varied greatly. This particular shelter was located in a church that had power and bathroom facilities (outhouse), but no running water. This meant that there were no showers, and no laundry facilities. All the refugees slept on cots and lived in a large open room that afforded little privacy. The DMH worker met with the couple and learned that their main concern was leaving the New Orleans area because they were both born in the area, and had never traveled very far from their home. Although they expressed their concern and stress regarding the prospect of staying in their current living situation at the shelter, they did not appear able to make the decision to move anywhere else. In discussing the situation they indicated that part of their stuck feelings of came from the difficulty in grasping the idea that their home was now gone. They kept listening to the news and hoping that things would change and perhaps they would be able to move directly back home. Unfortunately, each new report made it clear that this was not going to be possible in the near future. Almost all of their family and friends were located in the now flooded New Orleans area. Consequently, they struggled to find other family outside the storm affected area who would be able to provide housing for them.

One family member, who had been located and was willing to accommodate them, was in a northern part of the US. Interestingly the one concern they had about moving was the coming winter season. It was now September, and the move meant that they would soon experience their first snowy winter. They had little experience with snow, and the idea of a snowy winter was anxiety provoking for them both. The snowy environment symbolized this ultimate change that had occurred for them.

The DMH worker asked questions about this adjustment and what it meant to them in an effort to help them discuss each of their individual concerns and their ideas about the best path to take. This discussion included making a list of their concerns and encouraging them to talk about what more information they needed to make a good decision about next steps. The more they talked about it with the worker and each other the less anxious they became about the idea. Before, when the two of them tried to talk about it with each other, their anxiety would quickly rise and they found that they had gridlock in the discussion. In the end, they stated that they felt the DMH worker helped them by giving them a place to talk and express concerns without becoming too anxious. As each concern or issue came up, they discussed it openly and brainstormed about possible solutions.

Eventually they made the decision to make the move, but left open the option to return to New Orleans. They negotiated an agreement with each other that either one could call for a return to their home in the future, and that this would be accepted by the other partner without question. In the meantime they would do their best to make the move go smoothly. The more they discussed the move and prioritized their concerns and needs, the less anxiety they experienced. Towards the end of the discussion, the couple shared their spiritual convictions and how at times they felt that they had to turn over control to a higher power. The couple discussed other faith-based stories about migration and found comfort in thinking about this connection.

This case highlights several examples of how strategies from walk-in single-session therapy can be helpful in the DMH setting. First, the therapist accepted the client concern at face value and worked to help them prioritize their goals. The intervention focused on only providing the help that was requested, and was oriented to use the clients' own natural strengths and resiliencies (spiritual convictions; couple support system). The one small step that they felt would help them begin the process of moving forward was the agreement to move back to New Orleans if they chose. This seemed to free them to see more options in the situation and lowered their anxiety about making the next move.

Case Example #2: Give and Take

One DMH worker was stationed at a food distribution center at the center of a small town that had both been hit by the storm and had accepted a large number of refugees from the New Orleans area. Many of the little towns surrounding New Orleans saw their populations effectively double after the storm. At the same time, their own citizens struggled with blocked roadways, loss of power, lack of water, and scarcity of basic services. The loss of power meant that there was no air conditioning; the heat inside homes could exceed 100 degrees in the daytime. The food distribution centers became one of the main community hubs that many people would visit several times a day. DMH workers in this center would help serve the food, while also being available for those who may request counseling support.

Most people ate the meals in the large makeshift cafeteria that was provided, because it was powered by generators and was one of the few places that had air conditioning in the town. The DMH worker observed that one senior man came each mealtime and collected two meals to take away.

One day the man approached the DMH worker and asked if they could talk about a concern he had about his wife. He explained that the extra meal was for her, and that she would come with him each day to collect it. However, she would not get out of the car that he always parked a distance away because she did not want to be seen. The husband told the worker that he was worried that she was becoming progressively more depressed. When the volunteer asked what he felt was the main cause of her depression, the husband reported that his wife had always seen herself as a leader and "giver" in the community. He said this had provided her a special sense of pride that was now missing. He thought she was becoming more and more ashamed and reclusive because she was required to take food and other support from aid organizations. The husband reported that she more frequently stayed inside their home, which was without power and was badly damaged from fallen trees blown down by the high winds that came through the area. The husband believed that if his wife would "just get out more she would feel better, but instead she hardly ever went out now." The husband thought that if the DMH worker would come out to his car and "talk some sense into her" that she might not feel so ashamed.

When the DMH volunteer met the woman at her car, she openly discussed her sadness about what had happened with the storm and how helpless she felt she had become. She wanted to help all the other people who had evacuated, but said she worried that she was not even able to help herself. They discussed her background and the ways that she had been able to help her community in the past. She said that she had herself worked to provide food for the needy of her town. With some pride she said that she was an organizer and that she also enjoyed cooking. As she recounted her history providing food to those in need, her energy picked up and she smiled a bit as she told the volunteer about her own past aid work. He asked if she would feel better about things if she was able to do something to help the community.

After some discussion with the kitchen manager, the counselor approached the wife and asked if she could help serve food in the kitchen complex. He explained that he had spoken with the kitchen manager and that they were short handed and could use some help, especially from someone who knew the people in the area and had experience in food service work. The wife smiled widely and said she would be happy to help and was ready to start anytime. Soon both the husband and wife began serving food in the kitchen complex. Her depressive symptoms vanished, and she became a central person in the food distribution center, greeting those who came by name with a big smile.

This case example highlights several elements of single-session strategies in a DMH setting. Again, in this situation the worker accepted the client's concerns and goals at face value and provided only the help that was needed. Key to helping these clients was the ability to utilize an existing strength or resource. Fortunately, the client's resource also proved to be a resource for the community.

Caring for the Helpers, Self Care and the Unique DMH Setting

The massive influx of people from New Orleans to the surrounding towns created a small secondary crisis that required special consideration and sensitivity. Housing was in short supply and most aid workers slept in makeshift shelters that provided little or no privacy and often lacked showers and other basic comforts. Some aid workers, not wanting to take up space that could be used by others, brought tents and camped where they could find space. In this context an important part of the DMH workers' job was to provide counseling for the other helpers. This involved making sure aid workers attended to their own needs, took breaks from their work, slept at regular intervals, called home to connect with family, and dealt with their own vicarious traumatization associated with the aid work.

In my experience with walk-in single-session therapy I have observed that one of the main limitations of the work can be the mindset of the therapists doing the work. Because most therapists are trained in traditional clinical service delivery practices (outpatient, weekly, ongoing, regular meetings) a single-session practice requires some adjustment. At times this adjustment involves overcoming the therapist's preconceptions about the nature of clinical service delivery and change. They often must broaden their perspective to the possibility that, in some situations, many people can be substantially helped in one meeting. One of the foundational tenants of the ancient Greeks was to "know thyself" as a starting place in the pursuit of knowing others. Therefore, therapists benefit from some self-evaluation regarding their sense of how well they will work in this environment. Questions that a therapist may consider before beginning this work include: *How hopeful am I that meaningful change can be generated from a single-session meeting? How does working from a single-session perspective challenge my own beliefs about the nature of people and change? In what ways might my own beliefs hamper my efforts to help people in this type of work?*

I would like to share some thoughts for those who are considering applying walk-in single-session principles to the challenging, demanding, and, at times, heartbreaking work of disaster mental health counseling. This work is not for everyone, and it is important to consider your own level of comfort for working in this environment before you begin. During my deployment I met with many DMH workers who had been on several previous deployments and had accumulated some tips for those considering the job (Miller, 2006). These included:

- Before your deployment, make sure you will be able to endure the hardships of the assignment. If you know you would have difficulty with limited accommodations, it is better to pass on the assignment and look to provide help in other ways. Assess your own personal resources and your ability to respond to the needs of the deployment.

- When on deployment make sure to maintain some kind of schedule of sleeping and eating. The work can be arduous, but I observed that the dilemma was not getting workers to do the work, but getting them to stop when they were exhausted. There is always something that needs to be done in a disaster area. Without some schedule workers can find that they forget to sleep and eat. As the DMH worker, part of your job is to assess if the other workers are overworked or doing enough to take care of themselves. One usual first question I would ask other workers was when they last ate or slept. Often they were overdue for one or both.

- Find out the chain of command early in your assignment and follow it throughout your deployment. A national disaster area is naturally a place of chaos and confusion. Failing to follow the chain of command will only contribute to the chaos and make things worse. One of the main complaints from workers in a disaster area is the bureaucracy required to get some things done, but avoid the temptation to work outside the system.

- When on deployment, prepare to "hurry up and wait" for many of your daily tasks. You will need to be flexible with the organization and your fellow workers. As the DMH worker, you are often the one who works to calm the other workers down when they are frustrated regarding the delays and uncertainty that comes along with the job.

- While on deployment make sure to call home and connect with friends and family. It will be important for you to maintain your own resources, but it is also important for them to know how you are doing and that you are safe.

- Remember the importance of "out-processing" at the end of your deployment. Out-processing is your chance to tell your story about your experiences on the deployment; it will provide you with important closure. This process is analogous to the postsession discussion that occurs with the supervisor or team after a single-session meeting in situations where a team or supervision support is included. For some, it is difficult to disconnect from the work when it is time to go home. The DMH worker is the one who usually does the out processing session with the rest of the workers when they conclude their tour. This may seem like a minor part of the work, but I learned that it is a very important process. Many workers have experienced traumatic and difficult events and, when they return home, they may have limited opportunity to discuss what they have seen with others who can relate.

Concluding Thoughts for Walk-In Single-session Work in a DMH Setting

Walk-in, single-session therapies have developed rapidly over the past two decades. As is true of any clinical modality, it is not a solution for all situations. Yet, as Marshal McLuhan (1964) tells us, sometimes "the medium is the message." In some situations a single-session walk-in service communicates to the public that not all problems that therapists treat require invasive, costly, long-term treatments. The medium communicates that, for some situations, the natural resiliencies and capacities of people are the most important part of healing, and that the therapist serves as a catalyst—versus the origin—for change. The therapist is in the role of consultant for change, not the provider of change. Continued research is needed to determine when this medium of therapy is most useful, and when it may get in the way of change. For now it is clear that walk-in single-session approaches have great promise in the future development of a coordinated, multi-level response to disaster mental health treatments.

My work with the American Red Cross in Louisiana was the most challenging, yet rewarding work of my career. As my term of deployment ended, I found I was exhausted and ready to go home, yet also reluctant to disengage from the people of Louisiana. As fate would have it, I was traveling out the day hurricane Rita was making landfall. I observed many people panic in the airport, desperately trying to gain passage to sold-out flights. Part of me wanted to keep working and continue helping, but in the end I knew that I would need to heed the advice I had given to others—to know my limits and to let go when it was time to go home.

In this chapter I have endeavored to show how the lessons learned from traditional walk-in single-session therapy can be used in a variety of other settings, such as DMH services. This work is one step towards meeting the challenge made by Ignatio Martín-Baró, the father of the liberation psychology movement. His admonishment to our field was to revise our work from the bottom up (from our basic premises) and explore how to help people not only from our offices, but also from the environment in which people live, and struggle to live. This revision must continually look to serve those who may need us the most, not just those who come knocking at our doors. Walk-in single-session therapy, and the principles that are foundational to this approach, provide one useful strategy in this direction.

References

Martin-Baro, I, A, Aron, S. Corne, & E, Mishler (1994). *Writings for a liberation psychology.* Harvard University Press.

McLuhan, M. (1964). *Understanding media: The extensions of man* (1st Ed.) McGraw Hill, NY, 1964; reissued MIT Press, 1994, with introduction by Lewis H. Lapham; reissued by Gingko Press, 2003

Berg, I, K. (1989). Of visitors, complainants, and customers: Is there really such a thing as resistance? *The Family Therapy Networker, 13(1),* 21-25.

Bobele, M., Miller, J. K. & Slive, A. (2009). *Walk in single-session therapy: A systemic response to national disaster.* Paper presented at the American Family Therapy Academy (AFTA) Annual Conference. New Orleans, LA.

deShazer, S. (1988). *Clues: Investigating solutions in brief therapy.* New York: W. W. Norton & Co.

Hoffart, B., & Hoffart, I. (1994). *Program evaluation of the Eastside Family Center.* Unpublished manuscript.

Hubble, M.A., Duncan, B. L., & Miller, S. D. (Eds.) (1999). *The heart and soul of change: What works in therapy.* Washington, D.C.: American Psychological Association.

Jacobs J., Horne-Moyer H. L., Jones R. (2004). The effectiveness of critical incident stress debriefing with primary and secondary trauma victims. *International Journal of Emergency Mental Health 6 (1):* 5–14.

Kagee, A. (February 2002). Concerns about the effectiveness of critical incident stress debriefing in ameliorating stress reactions. *Critical Care, 6* (1): 88.

Miller, J. K., Banks, E., Goodwin, A., Fick, A., Froerer, A., & Stroyman, O. (2006, April). *The reluctant client: Breaking down the barriers to clinical service delivery.* Paper presented at the 2006 Annual Conference of the Oregon Association for Marriage and Family Therapy, Eugene, OR.

Miller, J. K. (2008). Walk-in single-session team therapy: A study of client satisfaction. *Journal of Systemic Therapies, 27,* 78-94.

Miller, J. K. (2006). First on the scene after disaster strikes: What to expect as a mental health worker. *Family Therapy Magazine, 5 (2),* 6-11.

Miller, J. & Slive, A. (2004). Breaking down the barriers to clinical service delivery: Walk-in family therapy. *Journal of Marital and Family Therapy, 30,* 95-103.

Miller, J. K. & Slive A, (1997). *Walk-in single-session therapy: A model for the 21st century.* Paper presented at the 1997 Annual Conference of the American Association for Marriage and Family Therapy, Atlanta, GA.

Miller, J. K. (1996). *Walk-in single-session therapy: A study of client satisfaction.* Dissertation: Virginia Polytechnic Institute and State University.

Minuchin, S. & Fishman H. C. (1981). *Family therapy techniques.* Cambridge, MA: Harvard University Press.

Mitchell, A. M., Sakraida, T. J., Kameg, K. (2003). *Critical incident stress debriefing: Implications for best practice. Disaster Management and Response.* Apr-Jun; 1(2):46-51.

Murray, C., & Lopez, A. (1996). *Global burden of disease: A comprehensive assessment of mortality and disability from diseases, injuries, and risk factors in 1990 and projected to 2020.* Boston: Harvard University Press.

Prochaska, J., & DiClemente, C. (1992). Stages of change in the modification of problem behavior. In Eisler, R., & Miller, P. M. (Eds.), *Progress in Behavior Modification,* (p.38). Sycamore, IL: Sycamore Publishing Company.

Rice, D. P., & Miller, L. S. (1996). The economic burden of schizophrenia: Conceptual and methodological issues, and cost estimates. In M. Moscarelli, A. Rupp, & N. Sartorious (Eds.), *Handbook of mental health economics and health policy. Vol. 1: Schizophrenia* (pp. 321–324). New York: John Wiley and Sons.

Slive, A., MacLaurin, B., Oakander, M., & Amundson, J. (1995). Walk-in single-session therapy: A new paradigm in clinical service delivery. *Journal of Systemic Therapies, 14* (1), 3-11.

Slive, A., McElheran, N., & Lawson, A. (2002). Family therapy in mental health centers: The Eastside Family Center. In M.M. MacFarlane (Ed.), *Family therapy and mental health: Innovation in theory and practice* (pp. 35-45). New York: Haworth.

Slive, A., McElheran, N., & Lawson, A. (2002). Family therapy in walk-in mental health centres: The Eastside Family Centre, in Macfarlane, M.M. *Family therapy and mental health: Innovation in theory and practice*. New York: Haworth.

U.S. Department of Health and Human Services. (1999). *Mental health: A report of the surgeon general—executive summary*. Rockville, MD: U.S. Department of Health and Human Services, Substance Abuse and Mental Health Services Administration, Center for Mental Health Services, National Institutes of Health, National Institute of Mental Health.

Walsh, F. (2006). *Strengthening family resilience*, 2nd ed. New York: Guilford Press.

Epilogue

Arnie Slive, Ph.D.
Monte Bobele, Ph.D.

In this book, we have shown that single sessions are a frequently occurring phenomenon and that even clients with long standing issues can be helped in one hour. For therapists to capitalize on this phenomenon, what is needed are alternative ways to think about single sessions—a different mindset. Some of these alternative views include the following:

- Clients know what is best for them. Researchers have established that clients often choose to attend one session of therapy. If some clients expect to attend therapy for only one session, then therapists must learn how to work with them and to celebrate that they have clients who are prepared to make the most of one therapeutic hour.
- Research evidence shows that most change occurs in the initial sessions of therapy. Why delay the inevitable? Let's get to work right away!
- When clients choose not to return for a second session, our best guess, based on research evidence, is that they chose not to return because they got the help they wanted in the first session.

We have also shown that walk-in counseling may be an effective way of providing self-contained single sessions of therapy. When clients do not have to jump hurdles to wait to be seen by appointment, they may be even more motivated to get on with things—to take immediate steps in a new direction.

In his concluding comments, John Miller (Chapter Ten) quotes Marshall McLuhan (1964): "The medium is the message." The fact that walk-in counseling services exist may promote the view that change can be facilitated in very brief therapeutic encounters and that such help is immediately available. The presence of walk-in services also communicates to mental health professionals that it is possible to form a collaborative therapeutic relationship in a very short period of time that produces rewarding results. We do not believe that walk-in counseling is the solution to all problems. We can only speculate about the impact of a walk-in service on a larger network of mental health services. Future research will help to decide where walk-in services fit into the larger mental health services picture. In the meantime, new opportunities arise for the development of walk-in services. In fact, since we began working on this book, we (Arnie and Monte) have been involved in two new walk-in counseling projects.

In Texas, the Austin Child Guidance Center (ACGC) began offering walk-in services to children, adolescents and their families as a way of reducing a growing waiting list. Offering walk-in services allowed ACGC to entirely eliminate their waiting list. Now, when prospective clients call to ask for an initial appointment, they are given an appointment only if a therapist has a slot available within two weeks. If no slots are available, they are told they can call back and try again or use the walk-in service. Most of the therapists who see the walk-in clients are volunteers who are either licensed mental health professionals or working on their licensing requirements. Clients who have used the walk-in service so far range in age from 6 to 16 and are usually seen with parents or guardians. Presenting concerns have included depression, anger, violence, suicidal ideation or self-harm, school avoidance, physical and sexual abuse, and anxiety problems such as OCD symptoms. For most, one session has been sufficient. For others, referrals are made to ACGC programs or to other community resources. All clients are invited to return to the walk-in service as needed.

In San Antonio, Haven for Hope is a new multi-partnered service for the homeless that opened earlier this year. It houses more than 800 people, both individuals and families. In addition to providing a safe place to stay it offers extensive mental health, medical and social services. In a partnership with Our Lady of the Lake University's Community Counseling Service (Chapter Seven), counseling is offered on site by appointment or by walking in. The intention is to focus on the most immediate issues facing the homeless so that they can get started on a new track. This is a fledgling project that we plan to report on in the coming months.

This book is a marking point in a journey that began for us when we met in Calgary in the early 1990's. While we each went our own ways in our walk-in and single-session work from there, in 2007 we were able to join up in San Antonio and have been working closely together since. We thank our colleagues and students in Calgary and San Antonio for their indispensable contributions to the ideas described in the book. We hope those ideas stimulate further thinking about the development of walk-in services as well as research regarding its impact and efficacy.

Now everybody's talkin' 'bout your new way of walkin',
Do you wanna lose your mind?
Lord, walk right in and sit right down, daddy, let your mind roll on.

References

McLuhan, M. (1964). *Understanding media: The extensions of man* (1st Ed.) McGraw Hill, NY, 1964; reissued MIT Press, 1994, with introduction by Lewis H. Lapham; reissued by Gingko Press, 2003.

Appendix A

THE FORMAT OF A WALK-IN SESSION

Presession

Clients walk in and are asked to fill out an intake form. The team reviews the form, selects therapist(s), and makes a preliminary plan.

The 20- to 30-Minute Session

Introductory Comments: "Here are a few things to fill you in on how we work, and then we can go from there. We offer services as a walk-in clinic, kind of like a medical walk-in clinic where you can come back again any time, though you may not see the same person again. When we're finished, I'll do a short write-up of this session so, if you come back again, we will have a record of what happened when you were here before. Some people find this hour is enough for them and some may like a referral for further services, and we can talk about that at the end. (*Note: Mentioning that some clients find one session sufficient plants a seed that one hour can work for them.*) The way this works is that we will meet together for about 30 minutes. I have colleagues behind the mirror who may phone in with a question for me to ask you. After 30 minutes I'll take a break and consult with my colleagues. Then I'll come back and share our collective thoughts. This way you have the ideas of multiple professionals."

The therapist then explains confidentiality and its limits.

A possible first question: "What are you hoping for in coming here today?"

- Engage and listen.
- What do the clients want from today's session?
- Set small goals.
- Highlight strengths, resources, exceptions, and what's helped in the past
- Ask contextual questions such as: "why now?", "what makes this a problem?", "who is involved in the doing and maintaining of the problem?"

We don't:

- Invite lengthy discussions about the past,

• Encourage speculation about why the problem exists, underlying cause, pathology, or unconscious motivations,
• Assume that insight produces change.

We do:

• Get descriptions of the problem in the present,
• Assume that "the problem is the problem" as presented by the clients,
• Focus on the problem as an aspect of human interaction,
• Establish specific goals described in behavioural terms,
• Assume that doing something different leads to change.

Intersession

The team discusses how the conversation has gone so far and whether a strong therapeutic alliance is developing. They indentify commendations and suggestions or ideas the therapists will share with the family. (Note: If no team is available, it is still recommended that the therapist take a "think" break.)

The 5- to 10-minute feedback to clients

• First, commend/compliment the clients based on the strengths and resources they described or you've observed.
• Second, ask if the session addressed what the clients wanted. This could involve simply asking if the clients had the opportunity they wanted to share their story. It could include a new way of thinking about the problem (a reframe). Or it could involve something new to try, to do, to experiment with as a first small step toward their goal.
• Third, discuss what's next for the client such as future walk-in sessions or a referral. Always invite clients to return for another walk-in session as needed.

The feedback part of the session should not be treated as the beginning of "Session 2."

The Team Debriefs

Appendix B

Sample Clinical Vignettes Discussed during MHWI Seminars

Context

MHWI staff meets quarterly for two hours. After the business meeting, they divide into three small groups and each group discusses a different vignette for 20 minutes. Then the whole team reconvenes as a large group to hear each other's conversation and share clinical approaches.

Vignette #1

A 12 year old comes to Walk-In by herself. She was told about walk-in by her school counselor. When the team reviews the form, the client's responses about risk and family violence are a little worrisome. What do you do?

(Please look at any policies/procedures that might be useful to you and share these with the whole team.)

- See the 12 year old by herself and then decide about parental involvement during the intersession break.
- The Shift Coordinator talks to the 12 year old in the waiting room. The young person is told she cannot be seen alone. She is invited to come back with her parent(s).
- Without the client's knowledge you call the parents to obtain consent before you meet with the client.

Vignette # 2

Sheila is 25. She presents to walk-in by herself with concerns about feeling down, lonely and unfocused in her life. She has recently moved here, she has a limited social network and her family is in Newfoundland. You and the team really like this client. Behind the mirror someone remarks "She seems so lost I just want to take her home for awhile and help her out".

During the break the team members have lots of ideas to offer such as resources, readings, courses and websites. You know this might be the only time this woman seeks help. But you wonder if "more I better?" or "is less better?"

- Please talk about your personal beliefs about how much information to provide a client with at the end of walk-in, a single session therapy.
- How do your beliefs mesh with the Eastside single session therapy model "More is not better, better is better" (Miller & Slive, 2004) Rather, the goal is to find out what the client wants and give him/her that. In this clinical vignette, is it possible that **our** desire to help may invite us to overlook what the client wants?

Vignette # 3

Sometimes family members do not particiapte in the therapy session, but the feedback from the family inovlement survey indicates that they are often very interested in the ideas and direction that are offered to the client by the team.

Please discuss ideas for talking to the client about how they might share information from the walk-in session with a family member who was in the waiting room or at home. Generate two concrete ideas/directions that a therapist could use.

About the Authors

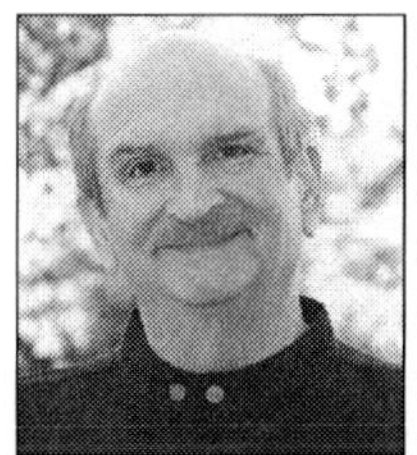

Monte Bobele, Ph.D. is a licensed psychologist and professor of psychology at Our Lady of the Lake University (OLLU) in San Antonio. He has been interested in brief therapies since completing a post-doctoral fellowship at the Galveston Family Institute in the late 1980's. He was one of the founding faculty members of the Lake's PsyD program in counseling psychology. He teaches graduate courses in systemic therapies and supervises graduate students in the department's Community Counseling Service, the Center for Miracles (a multidisciplinary service for abused children and their families), and The Haven for Hope a new comprehensive center for the homeless in Bexar County. He has also been involved in OLLU's development of a program designed to train culturally and linguistically competent psychologists to work with Spanish speaking populations. He frequently presents on brief therapy and multicultural training at national and regional professional conferences. He has co-led several immersion programs in México. He spends his spare time at his loom weaving or on his bike riding Texas' back roads.

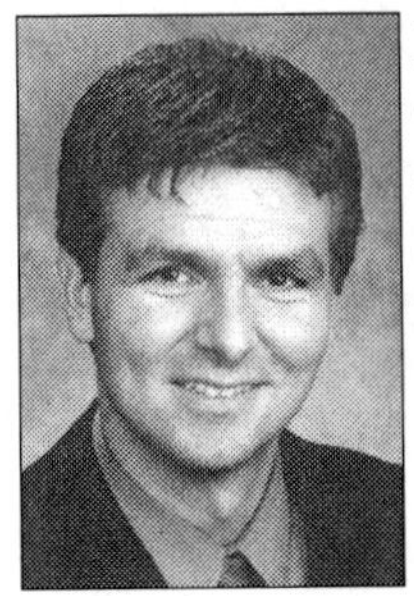

Ryan Clements MSW, RSW is a graduate of the University of Calgary Faculty of Social Work with a Masters in Social Work and is a registered social worker with the Alberta College of Social Workers. He specializes in clinical practice. Ryan has worked for Wood's Homes, a community based children's mental health centre, for 13 years and has held a number of senior leadership and clinical positions within the organization. Ryan's experience includes working with children, youth and their families in residential treatment settings related to exposure to domestic violence, adolescent sexual offenders, dually diagnosed adolescents with mental health issues, and community residential stabilization. Ryan is currently the Program Manager of the Wood's Homes community counseling and crisis services which includes the Eastside Family Centre and the Community Resource Team. He supervises graduate students in their clinical development. Ryan is also actively involved in Wood's Homes development of Outcome Based Service Delivery in partnership with the regional child welfare authority, and has presented the agency's work at various conferences, symposiums, and lectures.

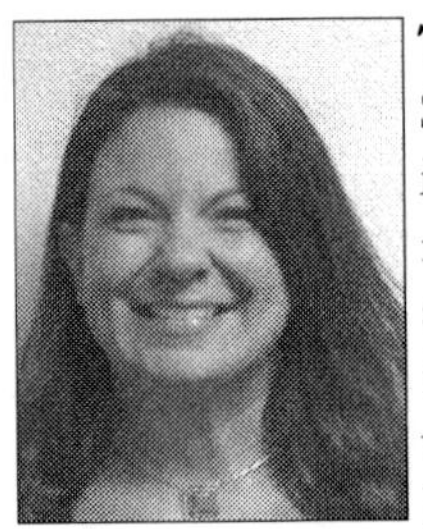

Teresa D Correia, MS, graduated from Southern Connecticut State University in 2004 with a degree in Community Counseling. She is a volunteer within the Pastoral Ministry of St. Patrick's Church in Colorado Springs, CO where she provides spiritually based counseling to homebound families and co-facilitates a grief support group. She is currently working toward a PsyD in Counseling Psychology from Our Lady of the Lake University and is interested in using brief therapies, particularly Single Session Therapy, to help families from underserved populations.

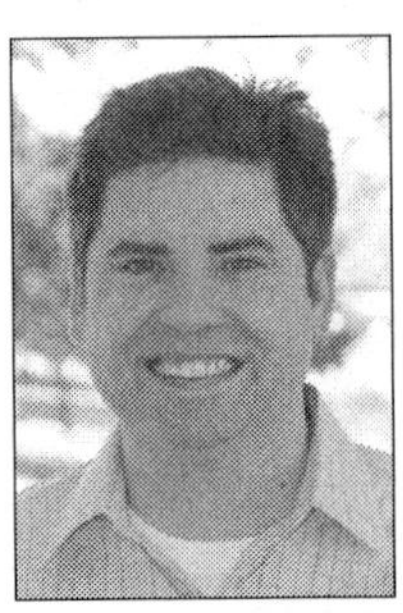

Kyle Green, MS, is a fifth year psychology doctoral student at Our Lady of the Lake University. Kyle supervises one therapy team at the Community Counseling Service and works part-time as a therapist-in-training at a local psychiatric hospital. His experience includes providing counseling and assessment services to families of children with disabilities, sexual assault survivors, combat veterans, clients with substance abuse, and walki-in counselling clients. Kyle has extensive training in multicultural competence and has worked with a diverse population of families, couples, and individuals.

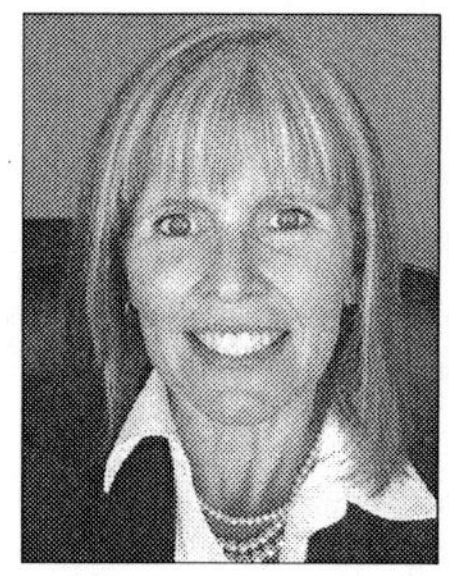

Lee Hackney, M.Sc. is a Registered Psychologist with the College of Alberta Psychologists who began her career working with children who lived on the edges of poverty and were spending much of their time on the street. This eventually led to work in clinical assessment and research in the areas of early development and attachment. For the past 12 years she has worked for Wood's Homes in a variety of programs that have included residential, school and community outreach. There she has been involved in working with families who have lived with abuse and attachment disruption as well as families that are struggling with mental health difficulties. She has written and presented on RBI: Relationally Based Interventions for front line workers, which speaks to the therapeutic nature of relationship in residential care. Lee has worked at Eastside Family Centre in different capacities for the last 13 years. She is currently the clinical coordinator of EFC where she provides therapy, and supervises students, interns and provisional psychologists. Apart from EFC, she teaches a course in lifespan psychology at a local university and is an examiner for the College of Alberta Psychologists.

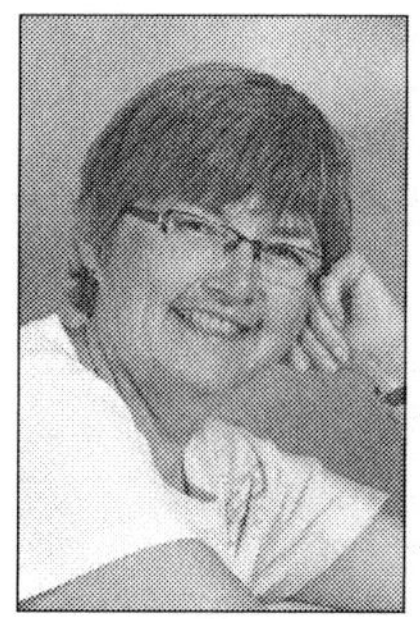

Sandy Harper-Jaques, RN, MN, RMFT is a clinical nurse specialist and clinical supervisor of two mental health outpatient programs at Alberta Health Services, Calgary. She is also a consultant to the Mental Health Nurses who work in an urgent care setting. Sandy is a member of the Canadian Nurses Association and a Clinical Member and Approved Supervisor with the American Association for Marriage and Family Therapy (AAMFT). Sandy's clinical work includes single-session walk-in therapy, provision of on-going therapy to adult clients, supervision, consultation and coordination. She is particularly interested in working with families where one family member has been diagnosed with a mental health problem. She also has a keen interest in the implementation of family nursing or family centered care into practice settings. Sandy has published on the following topics: family nursing, depression, single session therapy, commendations and anger and aggression. On a personal note, Sandy is married and has two daughters. Her daughters, now launched, are living in other cities.

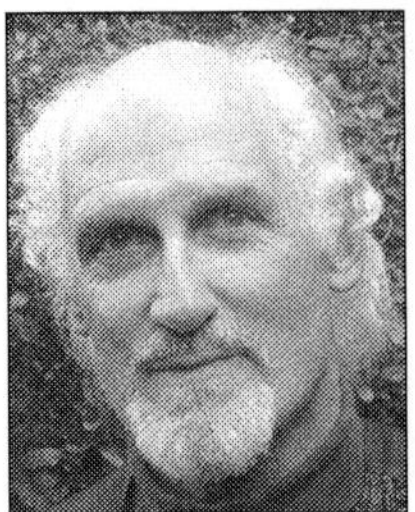

Michael F. Hoyt, Ph.D. (Yale '76) is a senior staff psychologist at the Kaiser Permanente Medical Center in San Rafael, California. He is the author of *Brief Psychotherapies: Principles and Practices*, *Some Stories are Better than Others*, *Brief Therapy and Managed Care*, *Interviews with Brief Therapy Experts*, and *The Present is a Gift*; as well as the editor of several volumes. He is a Woodrow Wilson Fellow and has been honored as a Continuing Education Distinguished Speaker by both the American Psychological Association and the International Association of Marriage and Family Counselors, as a Contributor of Note by the Milton H. Erickson Foundation, and was the 2007 recipient of the prestigious APF Cummings Psyche Prize for lifetime contributions to the role of psychologists in organized healthcare.

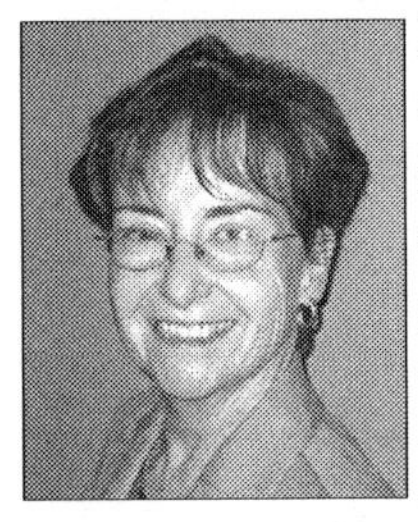

Maureen Leahey, RN, Ph.D. is a manager of mental health outpatient programs at Alberta Health Services, Calgary. She is an Adjunct Associate Professor in the Faculty of Nursing and Faculty of Medicine (Psychiatry) at the University of Calgary. She is a registered psychologist. Maureen is a member of the Canadian Nurses Association and a Clinical Member, Approved Supervisor and Fellow with the American Association for Marriage and Family Therapy (AAMFT). She was honored in 1997 and 2004 by AAMFT with the Organizational Contribution Award. In 2005, Dr. Leahey received the Distinguished Contribution to Family Nursing Award from the International Family Nursing Conference and the Journal of Family Nursing. Dr. Leahey is the co-author of five books including *Nurses and Families: A Guide to Family Assessment and Intervention*. It is in its fifth edition and has been translated into Japanese, French, Portuguese, Swedish, German, Icelandic and Korean. She is the co-producer of the "*How to" Family Nursing DVD Series* (www.familynursingresources.com). Dr. Leahey has written nine book chapters, twenty refereed articles and has delivered over sixty presentations at international conferences. Maureen's interests include brief therapy, family systems health care, supervision/training/consultation and work with larger systems.

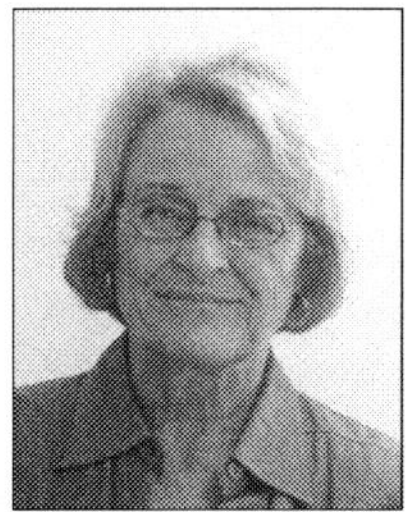

Nancy McElheran, RN, MN, RMFT is a clinical nurse specialist, approved supervisor with the American Association for Marriage and Family Therapy (AAMFT) and a clinical associate with the Faculty of Nursing, University of Calgary. Nancy's clinical interests are in the area of child/adolescent/adult and family mental health. Nancy worked at Wood's Homes, a community-based residential treatment facility for children, adolescents and their families with complex mental health needs for 17 years in both senior administrative and clinical roles. While at Wood's, Nancy was actively involved in the development of the Eastside Family Centre (EFC) Walk-in Counselling Service, the first of its kind in Canada, and in the development of the EFC Certificate Training Program for post graduate professionals in walk-in single session therapy. Nancy has presented the work of the Eastside in collaboration with her colleagues at international, national and local conferences and workshops. Her publications reflect her interest in walk-in single session therapy, mental health nursing and group therapy. Currently Nancy is in independent practice in Calgary, Alberta, is a consultant with Wood's Homes and is a board member with the Alberta Division of AAMFT.

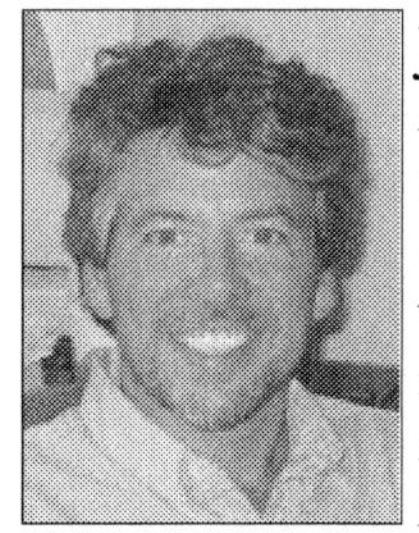

John K. Miller, Ph.D., LMFT is the Director of the *Sino-American Family Therapy Institute* and an Associate Professor in the Family Therapy Program at *Nova Southeastern University*. He is also a Fulbright Senior Research Scholar with the US Department of State (China, 2009-2010). His research interests include brief and time effective therapy models, innovations in clinical service delivery systems including walk-in single-session models, competency movement in couples and family therapy, and international family therapy (China and Southeast Asia). He has been traveling to Asia to conduct research and professional intercultural exchanges in psychology and family therapy since 2005. He has served as the president of the Oregon Association for Marriage and Family Therapy (OAMFT), and was elected to the board of the American Association for Marriage and Family Therapy (AAMFT) in 2009. He grew up in Louisiana and was trained in disaster mental health counseling after completing his graduate studies. He was a first responder in Louisiana after hurricane Katrina, working as a Disaster Mental Health Worker and Supervisor with the Red Cross.

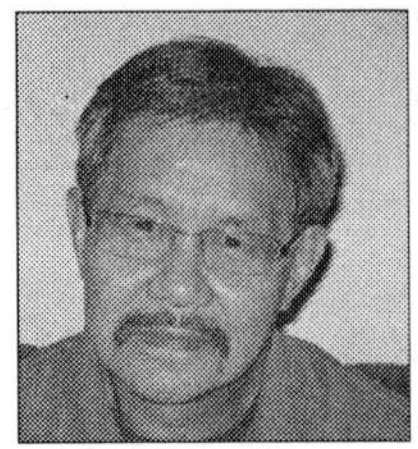

Harry Park, MSW, RSW is a Clinical Social Worker and Supervisor accredited with the Alberta College of Social Workers. He has been part of the Wood's Homes clinical service since 1990 working in community and residential programs. Harry was involved in the creation of the Eastside Family Centre (EFC) in 1990 and with the development of the Eastside clinical model. In addition to his own clinical practice, he has, from the inception of EFC, been a leader in the training of graduate students and post graduate professionals in the understanding and application of single session and brief therapy. He continues to offer training and supervision to graduate students, leads and develops a clinical team at EFC, and provides online teaching. Harry has presented on single and brief therapy locally and provincially. He also has an independent consultation and supervision practice. Harry was the first recipient of the Pulse of Social Work for excellence in clinical practice. He continues to be intrigued by the interplay between therapist and client systems. Current interests are the application of client focused practice to clinical practice, working with cultural change and domestic violence. He continues working with families with adolescents.

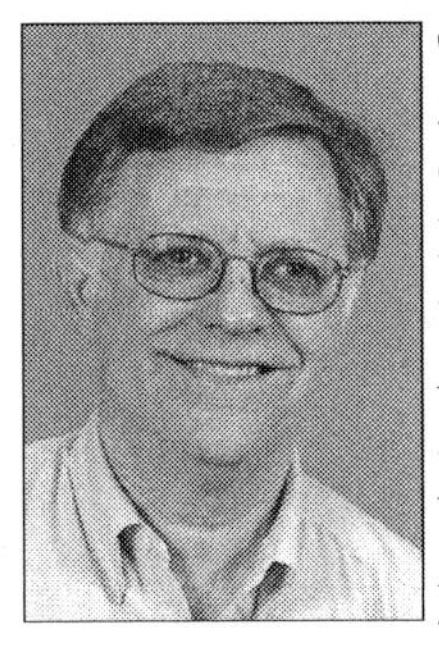

Gary R. Schoener is a Licensed Psychologist and since May 2010 Director of Consultation & Training for the Walk-In Counseling Center (Minneapolis). For 37 years he served as Executive Director of the Center. The center has received the American Psychiatric Association's Gold Achievement Award in Hospital and Community Psychiatry and other national recognition. A clinical psychologist by training, Gary was a member of the American Psychological Association's Advisory Committee on the Impaired Psychologist and its Task Force on Sexual Impropriety. He is the recipient of the Karl F. Heiser Award for advocacy in psychology as well as many other honors. The Royal Australia & New Zealand College of Psychiatrists chose him as their 2010 H.B. Williams Traveling Professor. He has lectured extensively in the United States and abroad. He is the senior author of *Psychotherapists' Sexual Involvement With Clients: Intervention & Prevention*, co-author of *Assisting Impaired Psychologists*, and many book chapters and articles. He has served widely as an expert witness in the US and Canada in cases involving professional practice standards, ethical violations, and sexual misconduct.

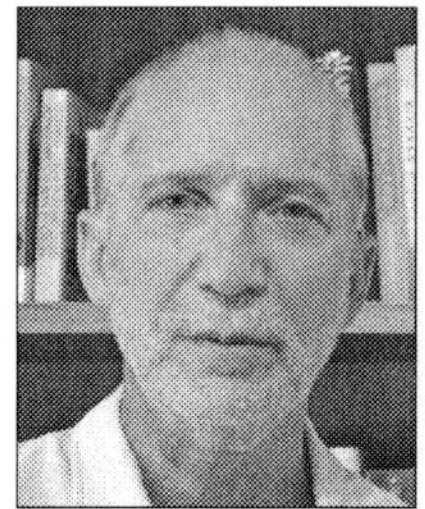

Arnie Slive, Ph.D. is a Licensed Psychologist (Texas) and Clinical Member and Approved Supervisor with AAMFT. His interests are in brief psychotherapy, program development, supervision and teaching. He has published in the areas of family therapy, residential treatment, adolescence, and single session, walk-in therapy. He formerly lived in Calgary, Alberta where he was a founder of the Eastside Family Centre and had a 20-year relationship with Wood's Homes as Clinical Director and consultant. He was a Clinical Associate Professor at the University of Calgary. He was past president of the Alberta Association of Marriage and Family Therapy. He is the recipient of the Divisional Contribution Award (AAMFT) and the Innovative Services to Family Award (Alberta Division, AAMFT). He now lives in Austin, Texas where he consults to community agencies and is a Visiting Professor at Our Lady of the Lake University (San Antonio). Arnie and Susan have been married for 42 years and are proud parents and grandparents.

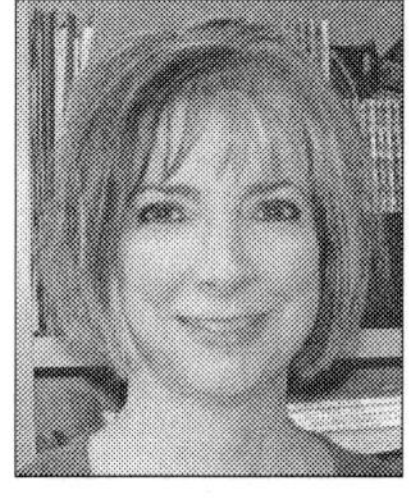

Karen Young, MSW, is a faculty member with Brief Therapy Training Centres International (a division of the Hincks-Dellcrest Institute) teaching in the Institute's Narrative Therapy Training Program and in the year-long clinical extern program in Brief and Narrative Therapy. She is the Manager of Clinical Services at Reach Out Centre for Kids in Burlington where she provides narrative supervision to staff and single session therapy services at the walk-in therapy clinic. She is a therapist with 27 years of experience working with children and families and has situated her therapeutic conversations within narrative practices for 21 years. Karen has provided narrative training and consultation to many agencies throughout Canada and assisted several to plan and initiate their own walk-in clinics. Karen has contributed numerous publications regarding the application of narrative therapy including papers published in the Journal of Systemic Therapies titled: *Co-composing an Evidence Base: The Narrative Therapy Re-visiting Project, From Waiting Lists to Walk-in: Stories from a Walk-in Therapy Clinic,* and *Narrative Practice at a Walk-in Clinic: Developing Children's Worry Wisdom.* Karen has a great deal of passion and excitement for narrative ideas and practices and is regarded as a trainer who conveys these ways of thinking and being in very clear and useable ways.

Index

NOTE: As both the theory and practice of walk-in, single-session therapy continue to evolve, many definitions and practices are anecdotal and change with the circumstance and location of the practice. To reflect the vibrancy of walk-in single-session therapy, this index lists key concepts both singly and as practiced in the six clinical situations described in the book.
Authors who are simply cited in this work are listed in Italics.